新医科英语系列教材

TRADITIONAL CHINESE MEDICINE & WESTERN MEDICINE
ENGLISH READING COURSE
VOLUME TWO

中西医英语
阅读教程

第二册

总主编◎云 红

主 编◎王良兰

副主编◎任忠勤
　　　　景先平

编 者◎余 凌
　　　　张 诣
　　　　梅宁琛

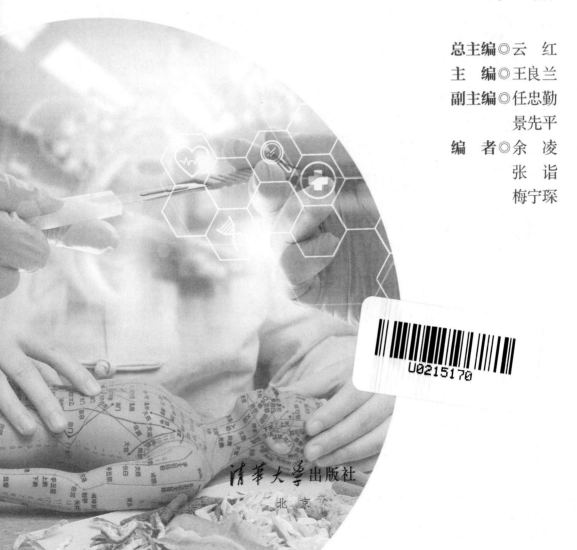

U0215170

清华大学出版社
北 京

内 容 简 介

《中西医英语阅读教程 第二册》共八个单元，每个单元由四部分组成：Pre-reading、In-reading、Post-reading、Additional Reading。Pre-reading 是单元的主题导入部分，旨在引导学生对主题进行思考，为接下来的课文阅读做好铺垫。In-reading 包含 Text A 和 Text B 两篇精选课文，旨在全方位提高学生的英语阅读理解能力；配套练习既能考查学生的语言基本功，又能检测学生在阅读实践中获取关键信息的能力。Post-reading 是一篇与主题相关的快速阅读文章，目的是训练学生利用已有阅读技巧准确、快速、有效地获取所需信息的能力；学生可以记录阅读时间和答题的准确率，自我诊断快速阅读能力的不足之处。Additional Reading 是课堂阅读的拓展和有益补充，学生可以根据自己的学习时间和英文水平有选择性地进行阅读。

本教材配有优质音频资源，学生可直接扫码听音。此外，本教材还配有参考答案，学生可登录 ftp://ftp.tup.tsinghua.edu.cn/ 下载使用。

图书在版编目（CIP）数据

中西医英语阅读教程. 第二册 / 云红总主编; 王良兰主编. —北京：清华大学出版社，2021.8
（2025.1重印）
新医科英语系列教材
ISBN 978-7-302-58131-4

Ⅰ. ①中… Ⅱ. ①云… ②王… Ⅲ. ①中西医结合－英语－阅读教学－教材 Ⅳ. ①R2-031

中国版本图书馆 CIP 数据核字（2021）第 086290 号

责任编辑：白周兵
封面设计：张伯阳
责任校对：王凤芝
责任印制：刘 菲

出版发行：清华大学出版社
    网　　址：https://www.tup.com.cn，https://www.wqxuetang.com
    地　　址：北京清华大学学研大厦 A 座　　　邮　编：100084
    社 总 机：010-83470000　　　　　　　　邮　购：010-62786544
    投稿与读者服务：010-62776969，c-service@tup.tsinghua.edu.cn
    质量反馈：010-62772015，zhiliang@tup.tsinghua.edu.cn
印 装 者：三河市铭诚印务有限公司
经　　销：全国新华书店
开　　本：185mm×260mm　　　印　张：10.75　　　字　数：182 千字
版　　次：2021 年 8 月第 1 版　　　　　　　　印　次：2025 年 1 月第 5 次印刷
定　　价：58.00 元

产品编号：092200-01

前　言

编写宗旨：

教育部高等学校大学外语教学指导委员会于 2020 年 10 月发布了最新的《大学英语教学指南（2020 版）》（以下简称《指南》）。《指南》在给大学英语课程定位时，提出能力、素质与素养导向；在给大学英语课程定性时，增加加深对中国文化的理解、服务中国文化对外传播的要求；在描述基于教学目标的大学英语课程设置时，增加"家国情怀和融通中外""一精多会""一专多能"等新要求。《指南》明确指出，大学英语课程应促进学生自主学习能力的发展和个性化学习策略的形成；进一步强调自主学习的重要性，明确学生在教学中的主体地位和教师作为组织者和引导者的角色；并且再次指出，大学英语教学兼具工具性和人文性的特点。《中西医英语阅读教程》以《指南》为指导，在设计、选材和编写中，力求准确把握大学英语教学的性质和目标。

《中西医英语阅读教程》以加强"新医科"建设为宗旨，以最新的中西医科普文章为素材，通过新颖的架构、针对性的练习以及开放式的讨论，着重培养学生的自主学习能力，夯实医学基础，增强跨文化交际意识，提高英语阅读能力。在增进西医知识的同时，了解中医文化。

理论指导：

《中西医英语阅读教程》的编写指导思想是批判性思维。罗伯特·恩尼斯认为批判性思维是指"为了决定什么可做、什么可信所进行的合理、深入的思考"。具有批判性思维的人能在辩论中发现漏洞，抵制毫无根据的想法。批判性思维绝非简单的否定性思维，它还具有创造和建设的能力，能够运用所获新知来解决社会和个人问题。批判性思维训练的目标是：寻找有效途径，训练这种能力。

这正是《中西医英语阅读教程》严格贯彻的理论基础。练习设计着重于有趣且富有思维挑战性的题型，如 Text B 的配套练习从以下几个方面训练批判性思维：（1）是否抓准"陈述"之意，即是否掌握每段大意；（2）判断推理是否清晰，即是否厘清各段的逻辑顺序;(3)判断"陈述"是否正确,即是否了解全文大意。编者希望以此种方式,循序渐进地训练学生的批判性思维。

教材特色:

1. 采用以内容为依托的(content-based)编写模式。本套教材较系统地介绍了医学基础知识,同时也能够增强学生的英语阅读能力。

2. 素材新颖,紧扣主题,语言地道、诙谐。本套教材对于广袤、错综复杂且神秘的医学森林,起到一个引导和桥梁的作用,吸引学生去探索这片神奇的医学森林。语料来源权威、专业,最大限度地提升选文的知识性、实用性和趣味性,激发学生的学习兴趣,使其能够学有所得。

3. 中西医结合,主题鲜明。选材兼顾中医和西医,中医相关内容以常见理念及治疗手段为主线,西医相关内容以器官系统为主线进行编排,学生从中可以较全面地学习医学基础知识。

4. 分级编写,难度恰当。本套教材既符合《指南》的要求,又参考词频的科学编排方法;运用科学、有效的软件,对每一篇拟选文章进行词频分析,在此基础上,再进行技术筛选、科学分级,帮助学生逐步提高英语阅读理解能力。

单元结构:

《中西医英语阅读教程》共分两册,每册八个单元。每个单元由四部分组成:Pre-reading、In-reading、Post-reading、Additional Reading。Pre-reading 是单元的主题导入部分,旨在引导学生对主题进行思考,由此及彼,触类旁通,为接下来的课文阅读做好铺垫。In-reading 包含 Text A 和 Text B 两篇精选课文,旨在全方位提高学生的阅读理解能力;配套练习既能考查学生的语言基本功,又能检测学生在阅读实践中获取关键信息的能力。Post-reading 是一篇与主题相关的快速阅读文章,目的是训练学生利用已有阅读技巧准确、快速、有效地获取所需信息的能力;学生可以记录阅读时间和答题的准确率,自我诊断快速阅读能力的不足之处。Additional Reading 是课堂阅读的拓展和有益补充,学生可以根据自己的学习时间和英文水平有选择性地进行阅读。从 Pre-reading 的编写到 Additional Reading 的设计,其背后的考量不外乎是最大限度地鼓励学生充分利用文本,做到学有所思,思有所得,得有所用,让阅读和思考成为一种习惯,并受益终身。

内容安排：

  本套教材内容分为两大板块：中医与西医。中医部分以常见理念及治疗手段为主线，西医部分以器官系统为主线，每一单元自成一个相对完整的内容体系。内容由浅入深，循序渐进。第一册为学生今后的英文医学文献阅读打下基础，中医部分主要由中草药、太极、针灸和艾灸组成；西医部分主要由心血管系统、呼吸系统、骨骼系统、肌肉系统、消化系统组成。中医话题是人们津津乐道的内容，西医中的这五大系统也是人们认知程度较高的内容，理解起来比较容易，故安排在第一册。第二册为提高阶段，中医部分主要由阴阳、五行、拔火罐和食疗组成；西医部分主要包括泌尿系统、神经系统、内分泌系统、被皮系统、生殖系统。这些内容较为抽象，学生只有具备更多的医学背景知识，才能更好地理解，因此安排在第二册。本套教材编排科学、合理，有利于提高学习效率。

  本套教材的编写团队来自重庆医科大学，具有丰富的一线英语教学经验，并且对医学有多年的接触和较深刻的认知。本套教材是我们多年教学研究和实践的结晶。在此，感谢老师们的支持和辛勤工作。所配图片选自 Pulse Hvvi、Shutter Stock、Verywell Health 等网站，在此对相关作者和网站表示衷心的感谢。

  限于编者的知识和阅历，教材中难免存在不足，恳请广大师生不吝批评指正。

编者

2021 年 5 月

Contents

Unit **1** The Urinary System

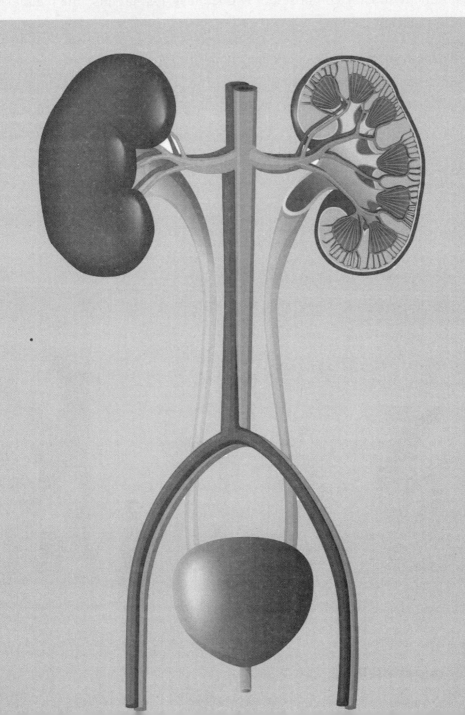

Pre-reading

The human body takes what it needs from food and changes it into energy. After this, waste products are left behind in the bowel and blood. The urinary system produces, stores, and excretes urine via a filtration mechanism in which potentially harmful molecules are removed from the body. It also plays a crucial role in water homeostasis, electrolyte and acid-base balance, and red blood cell production. The human urinary tract is comprised of two kidneys, two ureters, one bladder, two sphincters, and one urethra.

What can you do to help pass kidney stones? Do you know that your kidneys do a lot more than make urine? Can prostate cancer be prevented? Why do kidney patients face severe COVID-19 outcomes? The following passages may provide you with thought-provoking ideas.

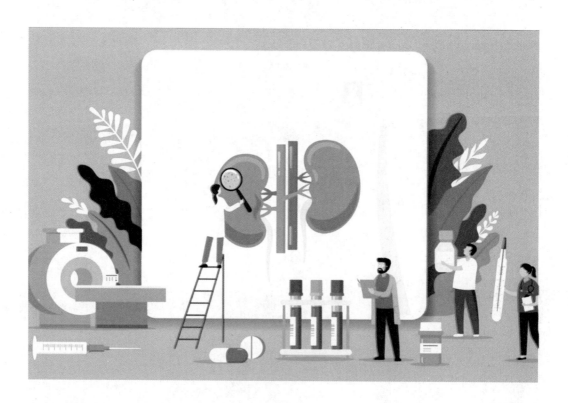

In-reading

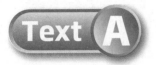

Five Things to Help Pass Kidney Stones

❶ If you've ever passed a kidney stone, you wouldn't probably wish it on your worst enemy, and you'll do anything to avoid it again. "Kidney stones are more common in men than in women, and in about half of people who have had one. Kidney stones strike again within 10 to 15 years without preventive measures," says Dr Brian Eisner, the co-director of the Kidney Stone Program at Harvard-affiliated Massachusetts General Hospital.

Where Do Kidney Stones Come from?

❷ Kidney stones develop when certain substances such as calcium, oxalate (草酸；草酸盐), and uric acid, become concentrated enough to form crystals in your kidneys. The crystals grow larger into "stones". About 80% to 85% of kidney stones are made of calcium. The rest are uric acid stones, which form in people with low urine pH levels.

❸ After stones form in the kidneys, they can **dislodge** and pass down the **ureter**, blocking

> **New Words and Expressions**
>
> **dislodge** /dɪsˈlɒdʒ/ *v.* to remove or force out from a position 离开原位；使……移动；驱逐
> **e.g.** The thorn of bone may dislodge from his throat without surgery.
>
> **ureter** /jʊˈriːtə/ *n.* either of a pair of thick-walled tubes that carry urine from the kidney to the urinary bladder 输尿管
> **e.g.** The scan showed a stone sitting across the left kidney's opening to the ureter.

New Words and Expressions

bladder /'blædə/ *n.* an organ that is shaped like a bag in which liquid waste (urine) collects before it is passed out of the body 膀胱
e.g. He has difficulty controlling his bladder.

urination /ˌjʊərɪ'neɪʃn/ *n.* the discharge of urine 排尿
e.g. The body discharges fluid through urination and sweating.

groin /ɡrɔɪn/ *n.* the part of the body where the legs join at the top including the area around the genitals 腹股沟
e.g. He's been off all season with a groin injury.

renal /'riːnl/ *adj.* of or relating to the kidneys 肾脏的，肾的
e.g. He collapsed from acute renal failure.

the flow of urine. The result is periods of severe pain, including flank pain (pain in one side of the body between the stomach and the back), sometimes with blood in the urine, nausea, and vomiting. As the stones pass down the ureter toward the **bladder**, they may cause frequent **urination**, bladder pressure, or pain in the **groin**.

❹ "If you experience any of these symptoms, see your primary care physician," says Dr Eisner. "He or she will likely perform a urinalysis and a **renal** ultrasound, an abdominal X-ray, or a CT scan to confirm kidney stones are the source of your pain and determine their sizes and number."

Let Kidney Stones Pass

❺ Stones typically take several weeks to a few months to pass, depending on the number of stones and their sizes. Over-the-counter pain medications, like ibuprofen (布洛芬) (Advil, Motrin IB), acetaminophen (对乙酰氨基酚) (Tylenol), or naproxen (萘普生) (Aleve), can help you endure the discomfort until the stones pass. Your doctor may also prescribe an alpha blocker, which relaxes the muscles in your ureter and helps pass stones more quickly and with less pain.

❻ If the pain becomes too severe, or if they are too large to pass, they can be surgically removed with a procedure called ureteroscopy. Here, a small endoscope (a device with a miniature video camera and tools at the end of a long tube) is passed into the bladder and up the ureter while you are under general anesthesia. A laser breaks up the stones, and then the fragments are removed.

Take Steps to Bypass Kidney Stones

7 Even though kidney stones can be common and recur once you've had them, there are simple ways to help prevent them. Here are some strategies that can help:

8 **Drink enough water.** A 2015 meta-analysis from the National Kidney Foundation found that people who produced 2 to 2.5 liters of urine daily were 50% less likely to develop kidney stones than those who produced less. It takes about 8 to 10 eight-ounce glasses (about 2 liters in total) of water daily to produce that amount.

9 **Skip high-oxalate foods.** Such foods, which include **spinach**, beets, and **almonds**, obviously raise oxalate levels in the body. However, moderate amounts of low-oxalate foods such as chocolate and berries, are okay.

10 **Enjoy some lemons.** Citrate (柠檬酸盐), a salt in citric acid, binds to calcium and helps block stone formation. "Studies have shown that drinking 1/2 cup of lemon juice **concentrate** **diluted** in water each day, or the juice of two lemons, can increase urine citrate and likely reduce kidney stone risk," says Dr Eisner.

11 **Watch the sodium.** A high-sodium diet can trigger kidney stones because it increases the amount of calcium in your urine. Federal guidelines suggest limiting total daily sodium intake to 2,300 milligrams (mg). If sodium has contributed to kidney stones in the past, try to reduce your daily sodium to 1,500 mg.

New Words and Expressions

spinach /'spɪnɪtʃ/ *n.* a vegetable with large dark green leaves that are cooked or eaten in salads 菠菜
e.g. Eat more carrots and spinach.

almond /'ɑːmənd/ *n.* a flat pale nut with brown skin that tastes sweet, or the tree that produces these nuts 杏仁；杏树
e.g. Today, almonds are still one of humankind's most beloved and healthiest nuts.

concentrate /'kɒnsəntreɪt/ *n.* a substance or liquid which has been made stronger by removing most of the water from it 浓缩物
e.g. Is the orange juice fresh or is it made from concentrate?

dilute /daɪ'luːt/ *v.* to lessen the strength or flavor of a solution or mixture 稀释，变稀薄；削弱
e.g. If you give the baby juice, dilute it well with cooled, boiled water.

⑫ **Cut back on animal protein.** Eating too much animal protein such as meat, eggs, and seafood, boosts the level of uric acid. If you're prone to stones, limit your daily meat intake to a quantity that is no larger than a pack of playing cards.

(667 words)

(Source: Solan, M. 2020. 5 Things that Can Help You Take a Pass on Kidney Stones. 01–29. From Harvard Health Publishing website.)

Task One

Decide whether the following statements are true (T) or false (F) according to the text.

1. _____ About 80% to 85% of kidney stones are made of uric acid.

2. _____ Kidney stones are likely to recur in most people who have had them.

3. _____ If kidney stones are too large to pass, they can be surgically removed with a procedure called ureteroscopy.

4. _____ The most useful way to prevent kidney stones is to drink a lot of water.

5. _____ Eggs are good for all people, including those who are prone to kidney stones.

Task Two

Fill in the blanks with the words and phrases given below. Change their forms if necessary.

intake	concentrate	dilute	depend on	procedure
trigger	dislodge	prescribe	prone	cut back

1. Sweeten dishes with honey, or _____ apple or pear juice.

2. The risk and severity of sunburn _____ the body's natural skin color.

3. Keeping a diary can help you work out your daily food _____ more accurately.

4. The physician may _____ but not administer the drug.

5. Richer countries must do more to _____ on carbon emissions.

6. The news raised eyebrows and questions about whether he was too old for the _____.

7. Water can _____ all kinds of chemical liquids.

8. After the dog got the ball, I tried to _____ it from her jaws, but I couldn't.

9. Old people's bones are more _____ to fractures.

10. When something important comes to an end, like a TV show or movie, it can _____ depression in some people.

Task Three

Paraphrase the following sentences from Text A.

1. If you've ever passed a kidney stone, you wouldn't probably wish it on your worst enemy, and you'll do anything to avoid it again. (Para. 1)

_____

_____

_____

_____

2. Over-the-counter pain medications...can help you endure the discomfort until the stones pass. (Para. 5)

_____

_____

_____

_____

3. If you're prone to stones, limit your daily meat intake to a quantity that is no larger than a pack of playing cards. (Para.12)

_____

_____

_____

_____

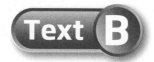

The Kidney Hormone that Helped Win a Nobel Prize

New Words and Expressions

accolade /ˈækəleɪd/ *n.* (formal) praise or an award for an achievement that people admire 赞扬，表扬；奖励，奖赏；荣誉

e.g. The Noble Prize has become the ultimate accolade in the sciences.

❶ Do you know that your kidneys do a lot more than make urine? Important in blood filtration and in balancing blood pressure, salt and acid levels, your kidneys also help make vitamin D, and a heroic hormone that alleviates altitude sickness and anaemia. Known as erythropoietin（促红细胞生成素）or "EPO", this hormone was the inspiration behind the highest **accolade** in modern medicine.

❷ It may be surprising that the kidneys can make a hormone controlling red blood cell production in the bone marrow, but that's exactly what the kidney hormone erythropoietin does.

Its production is exquisitely **attuned** to oxygen levels in the body and, under maximum EPO stimulation, the bone marrow can increase the rate of red blood cell formation tenfold—to 30 million per second. That's really helpful when you're at altitude, or if you suffer from anaemia.

❸ The decrease in density of air at altitude means that it contains less oxygen. Ascending Mount Kilimanjaro "too far and too fast", the medical physiologist Dame Frances Ashcroft recalls how her brain "slowly shut down through lack of oxygen". She describes staggering wildly, fighting for breath, and collapsing at the top of the crater rim with her head feeling as if knives were being driven through it and her vision swimming with black dots.

❹ Sensing this **hypoxia**, your clever kidneys release EPO, which comes to the rescue by boosting red blood cell production and so increasing the oxygen-carrying capacity of your blood.

❺ EPO is though quite slow at exerting its effects, getting to work within three to five days of arrival at altitude: ascend too fast and altitude sickness results; ascend too high, or for too long, and you risk your red cell levels becoming so raised that blood becomes thick and **viscous**. It is then harder for your heart to pump; heart failure may result.

❻ Injectable medications based on the EPO hormone have been manufactured, and have transformed the lives of thousands of people

> ### New Words and Expressions
>
> **attune** /əˈtjuːn/ *v.* to adjust or accustom (a person or thing); to bring into harmony with 使……协调
> **e.g.** Your angles want to help you attune your energies to higher frequencies.
>
> **hypoxia** /haɪˈpɒksɪə/ *n.* a condition in which not enough oxygen reaches the body's tissues 缺氧；低氧
> **e.g.** These signs of hypoxia are not dangerous in a healthy person.
>
> **viscous** /ˈvɪskəs/ *adj.* (of liquid) thick and sticky; not flowing freely 黏稠的
> **e.g.** Gases are much less viscous than liquids.

with advanced kidney failure, by treating their anaemia. Reflecting on their use in kidney failure, the consultant nephrologist Ashraf Mikhail describes how people changed from being "very pale, with no energy, and unable to walk very far" to those who "look healthy, go to work, and can take exercise even when they have advanced disease and are waiting for a **transplant**".

❼　Approximately 60% of people with solid tumors who have chemotherapy develop anaemia, since treatment can suppress the production of red blood cells in the bone marrow. The National Institute for Health and Care Excellence (NIHCE) recommends use of EPO-like drugs to treat the anaemia, since it can reduce the need for blood transfusions and lessen symptoms such as headache, **palpitations**, and shortness of breath.

❽　EPO has been termed Lance Armstrong's "drug of choice", having been one of a cocktail of supposedly performance-enhancing drugs that he took for years, before being stripped of his titles and medals. A subsequent study in athletes has shown that EPO may have **conferred** no athletic advantage at all.

❾　Blood doping through EPO injection (or through blood transfusion) has been used in sport with the illicit hope of boosting delivery of oxygen to an athlete's muscles through increasing the number of red blood cells in circulation. Between 1991 and 1994, the deaths of 18 young, otherwise healthy European cyclists were attributed to heart failure related to EPO abuse, writes Dr Frederic Martini, the denser blood placing an intolerable strain on the heart.

⑩ How exactly do cells in the kidney sense so exquisitely the low oxygen levels, prompting them to produce EPO? Hoping to **unravel** the molecular chain of events by which cells sense hypoxia, Sir Peter Ratcliffe, Professors William Kaelin and Gregg Semenza identified an entirely new system of **cellular** oxygen sensing—not unique to the kidney, but also found in the spleen, brain, and testes—that earned them the 2019 Nobel Prize in Physiology or Medicine.

New Words and Expressions

unravel /ʌnˈrævl/ *v.* to separate something 解开；拆散
e.g. I unraveled the string and wound it into a ball.

cellular /ˈseljʊlə/ *adj.* relating to cells 细胞的；由细胞组成的
e.g. Many toxic effects can be studied at the cellular level.

(643 words)

(Source: Cowan, H. 2021. The Kidney Hormone that Helped Win a Nobel Prize. 01–04. From Reader's Digest website.)

Task

Text B has ten paragraphs. Choose the correct summary for each of them from the list below.

List of Paragraph Summaries

1.	The kidney hormone EPO helped Sir Peter Ratcliffe, Professors William Kaelin and Gregg Semenza win a Nobel Prize.
2.	EPO, Lance Armstrong's "drug of choice", may have conferred no athletic advantage at all.
3.	Injectable medications based on the EPO hormone have been used in kidney failure.
4.	Blood doping through EPO injection has been illicitly used in sport.
5.	EPO gets to work slowly and heart failure may result.

6.	Ashcroft recalls what happened to her when she was ascending Mount Kilimanjaro.
7.	The kidney hormone EPO is really helpful when you're at altitude, or if you suffer from anaemia.
8.	Besides making urine, kidneys also help make vitamin D and EPO.
9.	Your clever kidneys release EPO in hypoxia.
10.	EPO-like drugs are recommended to treat anaemia.

Para. 1		Para. 2		Para. 3		Para. 4		Para. 5	
Para. 6		Para. 7		Para. 8		Para. 9		Para. 10	

Post-reading

Can Prostate Cancer Be Prevented?

New Words and Expressions

prostate /'prɒsteɪt/ *n.* an organ in the body of male mammals situated at the neck of the bladder that produces a liquid which forms part of semen 前列腺

e.g. Men over 55 should be regularly screened for prostate cancer.

❶ There is no sure way to prevent **prostate** cancer. Many risk factors such as age, race, and family history can't be controlled. But there are some things you can do that might lower your risk of prostate cancer.

Body Weight, Physical Activity, and Diet

❷ The effects of body weight, physical activity, and diet on prostate cancer risk aren't completely clear, but there are things you can do that might lower your risk.

❸   Some studies have found that men who are overweight or obese have a higher risk of developing advanced prostate cancer or prostate cancer that is more likely to be fatal.

❹   Although not all studies agree, several have found a higher risk of prostate cancer in men whose diets are high in dairy products and calcium.

> ### New Words and Expressions
>
> **selenium** /sɪˈliːnɪəm/ *n.* the chemical element of the atomic number 34; a gray crystalline non-metal with semiconducting properties 硒
> **e.g.** Experts say selenium plays a key role in the health of skin cells.

❺   For now, the best advice about diet and activity to possibly reduce the risk of prostate cancer is to:

- Get to and stay at a healthy weight.

- Keep physically active.

- Follow a healthy eating pattern, which includes a variety of colorful fruits and vegetables and whole grains, and avoids or limits red and processed meats, sugar-sweetened beverages and highly processed foods.

❻   It may also be sensible to limit calcium supplements and not to get too much calcium in the diet. (This does not mean that men who are being treated for prostate cancer should not take calcium supplements if their doctors recommend them.)

Vitamin, Mineral, and Other Supplements

❼   Vitamin E and **selenium**: Some early studies suggested that taking vitamin E or selenium supplements might lower prostate cancer risk.

❽   But in a large study known as the Selenium and Vitamin E Cancer Prevention Trial, neither vitamin E nor selenium supplements were found to lower prostate cancer risk. In fact, men in the study taking the vitamin E supplements were later found to have a slightly higher risk of prostate cancer.

⑨ Soy and isoflavones: Some early research has suggested possible benefits from soy proteins in lowering prostate cancer risk. Several studies are now looking more closely at the possible effects of these proteins.

⑩ Taking any supplements can have both risks and benefits. Before starting vitamins or other supplements, talk with your doctor.

Medicines

⑪ Some drugs might help reduce the risk of prostate cancer.

⑫ 5-alpha reductase is an enzyme in the body that changes testosterone（睾酮）into dihydrotestosterone (DHT)（双氢睾酮）, the main hormone that causes the prostate to grow. Drugs called 5-alpha reductase inhibitors such as finasteride（非那雄胺）and dutasteride（度他雄胺）, block this enzyme from making DHT. These drugs are used to treat benign prostatic **hyperplasia** (BPH), a non-cancerous growth of the prostate.

⑬ Large studies of both of these drugs have been done to see if they might also be useful in lowering prostate cancer risk. In these studies, men taking either drug were less likely to develop prostate cancer after several years than men getting an inactive placebo.

⑭ These drugs can cause sexual side effects such as lowered sexual desire and erectile **dysfunction** (impotence), as well as the growth of breast tissue in some men. But they can help with urinary problems from BPH such as trouble urinating and leaking urine (**incontinence**).

⑮ These drugs aren't approved by the FDA specifically to help prevent prostate cancer, although doctors can prescribe them "off label" for this use. Right now, it isn't clear that taking one of these drugs just to lower prostate cancer risk is very helpful. Still, men who want to know more about these drugs should discuss them with their doctors.

⑯ Some research suggests that men who take a daily aspirin might have a lower risk of getting and dying from prostate cancer. But more research is needed to show if the possible benefits outweigh the risks. Long-term aspirin use can have side effects, including an increased risk of bleeding in the digestive tract. While aspirin can also have other health benefits, at this time most doctors don't recommend taking it just to try to lower prostate cancer risk.

⑰ Other drugs and dietary supplements that might help lower prostate cancer risk are now being studied. But so far, no drug or supplement has been found to be helpful in studies large enough for experts to recommend them.

(688 words)

(Source: Anon. 2020. Can Prostate Cancer Be Prevented?. 06–09. From American Cancer Society website.)

Your reading time: _____ mins

Your reading rate: _____ words/min

Task

Read the text as quickly as you can and then choose the best answer to each question.

1. Which of the following might not help you lower the risk of prostate cancer?

   A. To get to and stay at a healthy weight.

   B. To follow a healthy eating pattern, which includes a variety of colorful fruits and vegetables and whole grains.

   C. To take as many calcium supplements as possible.

   D. To keep physically active.

2. Which of the following statements is not true about 5-alpha reductase inhibitors?

   A. They block 5-alpha reductase from making dihydrotestosterone.

   B. Both finasteride and dutasteride are inhibitors.

   C. These drugs can cause sexual side effects as well as the growth of breast tissue in some men.

   D. These drugs are used to treat prostate cancer.

3. What does "off label" in Para. 15 refer to according to your understanding?

   A. Being used in ways for which it has not been approved.

   B. Being unqualified.

   C. Being illegal.

   D. Being under test.

4. What is the surest way to prevent prostate cancer?

   A. To take aspirin.   B. To take 5-alpha reductase inhibitors.

   C. To take vitamins or other supplements.   D. None.

5. What is the purpose of the text?

   A. To recommend people some drugs and dietary supplements.

   B. To introduce people some things they can do to lower the risk of prostate cancer.

   C. To emphasize the importance of a healthy lifestyle.

   D. To convince people that prostate cancer can be prevented.

Your comprehension rate: _____ %

Additional Reading

Kidney Disease Death Rates in COVID Patients

❶   COVID-19 patients who have chronic kidney disease (CKD) or develop coronavirus-related kidney injury in the intensive care unit (ICU) face higher odds of death than their otherwise-healthy peers, according to a study published late last week in *Anaesthesia*.

❷   Led by researchers at Imperial College London, the **retrospective** study involved 372 adult COVID-19 patients in four ICUs in the United Kingdom from March 10 to July 31. Of the 372 patients, 216 (58%) had kidney impairment, 22% of which was CKD (48 patients) and 78% of which developed during hospitalization (168 patients).

Degree of Injury, Need for Dialysis

❸   In total, 139 of 372 patients (37%) died. Of the 156 patients with healthy kidneys, 32 (21%) died in the hospital, in contrast with 81 of 168 patients (48%) with newly developed kidney injury and 11 of 22 (50%) with CKD stage 1 through 4.

❹   Among the other 26 patients who had CKD, 9 of 19 patients (47%) with end-stage renal failure (ESRF), who had already required routine outpatient dialysis, died. The death rate was the highest in CKD patients who had undergone kidney transplants [6 of 7 (86%)].

> **New Words and Expressions**
>
> **retrospective** /ˌretrəˈspektɪv/ *adj.* concerned with or related to the past 回顾的；可追溯的；怀旧的
> **e.g.** In 1946, Moore had his first foreign retrospective exhibition at the Museum of Modern Art, New York.

⑤ Death rates rose along with worsening kidney injury classified by Kidney Disease: Improving Global Outcomes (KDIGO) Classification. Of 157 patients with stage 0 (least) injury, 33 (21%) died, compared with those with more serious stages 1 to 3 injury [91 of 186 (49%)].

⑥ Those who died were more likely to have needed dialysis than survivors [64 of 139 (46%) vs 57 of 233 (24%)]. But once dialysis was started, death rates were not significantly different between survivors and non-survivors in patients with new kidney injury [39 of 82 (48%) vs 43 of 82 (52%)] or non-end-stage CKD [8 of 17 (47%) vs 9 of 17 (53%)].

⑦ Among 216 patients with kidney impairment, 121 (56%) needed dialysis in the hospital, and 9 of the 48 survivors who required dialysis for the first time in the ICU (19%) continued to need it after they were released, suggesting that COVID-19 may lead to long-term kidney impairment. Most patients [337 of 372 (91%)] required mechanical ventilation. Median Acute Physiology and Chronic Health Evaluation (MAPCHE) Ⅱ score was 15, with 0 the least likely to die in the ICU and 71 the most likely.

Vigilance, Intensive Care

⑧ The authors said that they were surprised that the death rate in patients with ESRF and on dialysis, who usually have poorer outcomes in many other illnesses, wasn't significantly higher than in those with less-serious CKD and coronavirus-related kidney injury. The finding, they noted, suggests that COVID-19 patients receiving dialysis—including those with ESRF—have a similar chance for survival as those with less severe disease or injury and thus should be considered for ICU care.

9 But the researchers cautioned that their results may have been subject to selection **bias**, in which some patients with ESRF who were too sick for admission to the ICU may not have been included in the study during the peak of the last UK COVID-19 surge.

10 Patients were, on average, about 60 years old. 72% of them were men, and 76% were black or Asian.

11 The authors said, "We don't know exactly why patients with impaired kidneys are more likely than others to die of COVID-19 but **theorize** that it could be because the virus causes inflammation of the kidney blood vessels, similar to how it inflames the lungs; the enhanced immune response ["cytokine storm" (细胞激素风暴)] triggered by the virus injures the kidneys; or multiorgan failure leads to kidney tissue death."

12 "Our data demonstrate that renal impairment in patients admitted to intensive care with COVID-19 is common and is associated with a high mortality and requirement for on-going renal support after discharge from critical care," the authors wrote. "Attention needs to be paid to patients with COVID-19 with any form of renal impairment and every effort made to prevent progression of renal injury in order to reduce mortality."

New Words and Expressions

bias /ˈbaɪəs/ *n.* a tendency to prefer one person or thing to another, and to favor that person or thing 偏见
e.g. Some institutions still have a strong bias against women.

theorize /ˈθɪəraɪz/ *v.* to believe especially on uncertain or tentative grounds 推理；建立理论或学说
e.g. By studying the way people behave, we can theorize about what is going on in their mind.

New Words and Expressions

utilization /ˌjuːtɪlaɪˈzeɪʃn/ *n.* the act of using 利用；使用

e.g. Volvo Cars has introduced waste management systems to minimize residual products and improve material utilization.

⑬ The researchers also remarked that patients who require dialysis in the hospital have a much lower survival rate than those who don't, which could have implications for resource allocation. "The impact on resource **utilization** is considerable, especially in a pandemic situation where resources may have to be rationed," they wrote.

(701 words)

(Source: Beusekom, M. V. 2020. Kidney Disease Tied to High Death Rates in COVID Patients. 10–19. From Cidrap website.)

Task

Read the text carefully and then complete the statements with appropriate words.

1. Asthma is a chronic disease caused by respiratory _____.
2. Flights are _____ to delay because of the fog.
3. After the child had been treated, and was being prepared for _____ from the hospital, Dr Myer talked to the parents about how they should care for the child at home.
4. Researchers at Imperial College London conducted a(n) _____ analysis of 372 cases of adult COVID-19 patients.
5. Extreme stress can _____ the development of the nervous and immune systems.
6. Buying Twitter would give Google a real-time social information service and _____ amounts of data.
7. The nation's infant _____ rate has reached a record low.
8. A(n) _____ in new home sales and a drop in weekly unemployment claims suggest that the economy might not be as weak as some analysts previously thought.
9. Acute liver failure is a medical emergency that requires _____.
10. The _____ of dying is higher for COVID-19 patients who have chronic kidney disease.

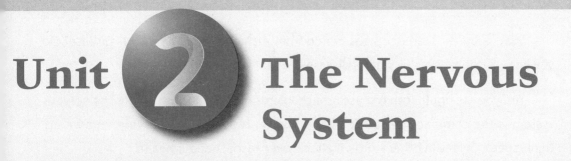

Unit 2 The Nervous System

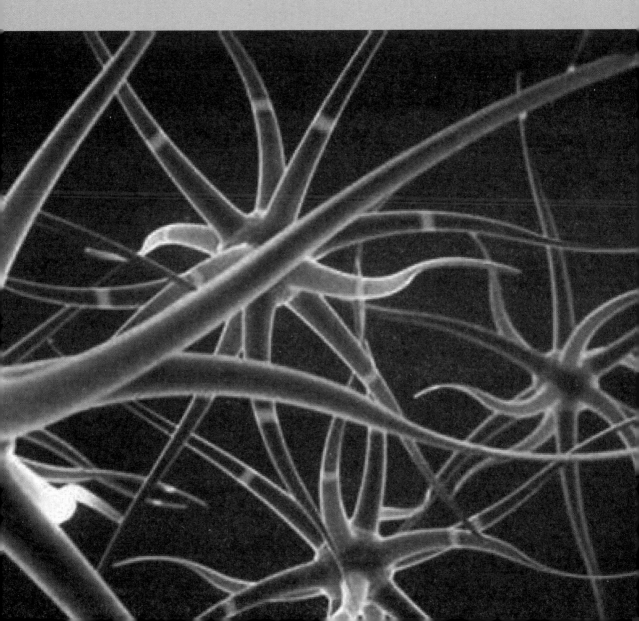

Pre-reading

Have you ever seen people suffering from Alzheimer's or Parkinson's disease? Do you know what causes this kind of diseases?

Yes, you are right! Both diseases are problems of the nervous system. The nervous system is the command center for our body, controlling almost everything we do, think, speak, or feel. In other words, it affects every aspect of our health.

How much do you know about the nervous system? Besides Alzheimer's and Parkinson's disease, are there any other diseases related to this system? Can these diseases be cured? What should the patients and caregivers do with the nervous system diseases? You may find out the answers in the following four stories.

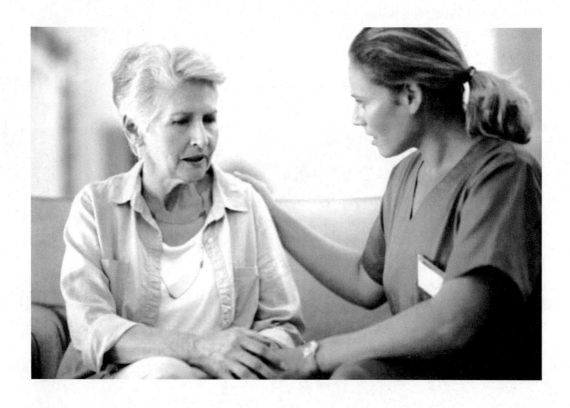

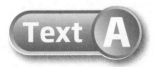

Alzheimer's Radically Changes the Lives of Patients

❶ Julie Burger of Vancouver, Washington, hid the initial symptoms of her dementia from her husband, Les. For more than two years, she had been losing her photographic memory, "slowly but surely", she says. Born in Puerto Rico, Julie speaks six languages and had been the **valedictorian** of her high school class. She'd earned a master's degree and served in executive and volunteer roles for the American Red Cross for half a century. All of this academic and professional success had been sustained by her incredible memory and her **voracious** appetite for the written word, so when her photographic memory started to slip and her rate of reading and level of comprehension dropped, she knew something was wrong.

❷ Her husband, Les, had been an internist, and he says he missed the early signs despite his medical training, because she hid her struggles so well. "Julie's the smart one in our family,"

New Words and Expressions

valedictorian /ˌvælɪdɪkˈtɔːrɪən/ *n.* the student with the best grades who delivers the speech at graduation ceremony（毕业典礼上）致辞的最优秀毕业生

e.g. My rival, who was the valedictorian after our neck-and-neck race for the top, taught me a lot of lessons.

voracious /vəˈreɪʃəs/ *adj.* excessively eager; having a huge appetite 如饥似渴的；贪吃的

e.g. Her appetite for information was voracious.

New Words and Expressions

thrive on to enjoy or be successful in a particular situation, especially one that other people find difficult or unpleasant（尤指在别人觉得困难的时候）以……为乐；可以出色地应对

e.g. Many people thrive on a stressful lifestyle.

he says. "She was able to keep this to herself, and I really wasn't aware of it until she came to me about four years ago and said 'something's wrong.'" By then, her mathematical abilities had slipped too.

❸ Once Les knew there was a problem, they went to see a doctor who diagnosed mild cognitive impairment. A year later, in 2016, Julie—then 76—had an amyloid PET scan（淀粉样蛋白 PET 扫描）that confirmed she had Alzheimer's disease. "I'd never heard the word Alzheimer's before," she says. But getting a diagnosis has enabled the Burgers to access treatment and helped them prioritize certain aspects of their lives. "Julie is still in the early phase of the disease," Les says, and while she retains some cognitive capacity, the couple are busy visiting as many family members and friends as they can. "She **thrives on** being with friends and family, and we're taking the time to visit them, mostly locally. The problem is that our world has gotten a lot smaller for both of us since she developed Alzheimer's," he says.

❹ Some of the smaller changes Alzheimer's has brought have been the hardest to cope with. "Julie doesn't remember our wedding. She doesn't remember the names of certain people. That's a lot more livable than the short-term memory problems. Literally from moment to moment, she puts something down and doesn't know where it is. When we're staying at someone's house, she can't remember where the bathroom is. She can't do finances at all and has no concept of time any longer and has trouble telling time. She can't follow a recipe. She can't make honey for the hummingbirds anymore."

❺ Les acts as Julie's primary caregiver, and though she sometimes tries to push him away out of frustration over what she can no longer do for herself, she's grateful for his support. "Les has been wonderful through this whole thing. He's my walking-talking Google. He's wonderful and he gets me to where I need to be."

❻ Julie is currently enrolled in a clinical trial of an Alzheimer's medication. Although they don't know whether the trial will make a difference in her case, the Burgers are clear-eyed about the need for further research and treatment options for others with the disease. As a doctor, Les says the anticipated rise in dementia diagnoses in America's aging population "reminds me of the time when we first learned about HIV/AIDS. There were those young people getting these incredibly bad infections and dying and we didn't have a clue. Here it is 35 years later and yes, we have treatments, but they're expensive. HIV/AIDS hasn't been got rid of, but it's better, and transmission rates in the US have declined. With Alzheimer's, we're in the same position. This big **tsunami** is coming, and we have to figure out how to deal with it and develop treatments. We have to see if we can halt this disease and cure it one day."

New Words and Expressions

tsunami /tsʊˈnɑːmɪ/ *n.* a very large wave, often caused by an earthquake, that flows onto the land and can cause widespread deaths and destruction 海啸

e.g. A terrible tsunami followed the earthquake.

(640 words)

(Source: Howley, E. K. 2019. Personal Stories from Dementia Patients. 06–17. From US News website.)

Task One

Decide whether the following statements are true (T) or false (F) according to the text.

1. _____ Julie Burger told her husband the initial symptoms of her Alzheimer's disease.

2. _____ Julie's academic and professional success was partly due to her good memory and reading.

3. _____ It had been more than three years before Julie's diagnosis of Alzheimer's disease.

4. _____ Julie has gradually lost her long-term memory but still keeps her short-term memory.

5. _____ We have known a lot about Alzheimer's disease, so it's quite likely that it will be cured soon.

Task Two

Fill in the blanks with the words given below. Change their forms if necessary.

slip	cognitive	tsunami	dementia	prioritize
thrive	valedictorian	anticipate	enable	voracious

1. The new test should _____ doctors to detect the disease early.
2. That new motivation made me a(n) _____ reader. In a two-year period, I had read over 150 books.
3. Make lists of what to do and _____ your tasks.
4. Another possibility is that children younger than three lack some _____ capacity for memory.
5. Creative people are usually very determined and _____ on overcoming obstacles.
6. There are pretty clear differences between signs of _____ and age-related memory loss.
7. The club had _____ to the bottom of Division Four.
8. More than 600,000 people were displaced by the _____.

9. That right path helped Slater navigate schools and neighborhoods, where gangs and drugs were the norms, to graduate as the class _____ at Gompers Academy.

10. The eagerly _____ movie will be released next month.

Task Three

Paraphrase the following sentences from Text A.

1. All of this academic and professional success had been sustained by her incredible memory and her voracious appetite for the written word... (Para. 1)

   _____

   _____

   _____

   _____

2. Les acts as Julie's primary caregiver, and though she sometimes tries to push him away out of frustration over what she can no longer do for herself, she's grateful for his support. (Para. 5)

   _____

   _____

   _____

   _____

3. This big tsunami is coming, and we have to figure out how to deal with it and develop treatments. We have to see if we can halt this disease and cure it one day. (Para. 6)

   _____

   _____

   _____

   _____

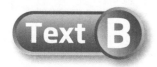

Waiting for the Other Shoe to Drop

New Words and Expressions

presentient /prɪˈsenʃɪənt/ *adj.* having a feeling that something will or is about to happen 有预感的
e.g. It's presentient that a snowstorm is coming.

adrenaline /əˈdrenəlɪn/ *n.* a chemical produced by your body when you are afraid, angry, or excited, which makes your heart beat faster 肾上腺素
e.g. There's nothing like a good horror film to get the adrenaline going.

❶ About five years ago, I first took notice of the trembling in my left hand. Indications might have taken place earlier, but as my wife and friends will tell you, I'm not the most observant of people.

❷ A little bit about me: I retired from the Air Force in 2004 and almost immediately earned my credentials and became a paid ski patroller at our local ski resort in Utah. My wife was a bit disappointed that I didn't take a more lucrative job in business. It may have been **presentient** when I told her I felt I had a narrow window of opportunity to do something requiring a certain degree of physical skill and I needed to take advantage at that point in time. Thank goodness, my wife accepted my desires, and the past 16 years have been filled with joy at my decision.

First Signs of Shaking

❸ But back to 2015, I was the first responder to an injured skier. As I worked on my patient, I noticed my left hand shaking. I completed providing the necessary care, packaged the patient into the sled, and saw him off, dismissing the shaking as a mixture of cold and the **adrenaline** rush of working on a patient. As time went on, so did the frequency. It took me two years before I brought the shaking to the attention of my doctor and his initial diagnosis was essential **tremors**, for which he put me on Primidone (普里米酮). The following year, during my normal wellness check, he noticed my **tumbling** while at rest and referred me to a neurologist. She diagnosed my condition as early stage of Parkinson's disease and placed me on a low dose of Ropinirole (罗匹尼罗).

④ That was 2018. I'm now at the maximum dosage allowable. I've been extremely fortunate, to date. I'm still functioning fairly normally… the left hand shaking is the most visible sign though my left foot is beginning to shake slightly at certain times too. I've noticed my sense of balance isn't what it was, though blaming it all on Parkinson's may not be fair since I am 68 now. Anyway, I'm still doing well enough to continue as a contributing member of the patrol though I have informed the Patrol Director of my malady, and have **recused** myself from participating in avalanche **mitigation** work for fear of not being able to support my partners in an avalanche situation.

Enjoying the Present Times

⑤ Life, for me, has remained pretty much what I would call: normal. I suffer very few side effects from the medication…the most telling are the sleep attacks which usually take place if I've had more than one alcoholic beverage (yes, I've fallen asleep while talking to my best friend and neighbor) or in the evenings while watching TV. I also find I can only sleep four

New Words and Expressions

tremor /'tremə/ *n.* a slight shaking movement in your body that you cannot control, especially because you are ill, weak, or upset（身体或声音的）颤抖；震颤
e.g. The medication can cause hair loss, tremors, and increased weight.

tumble /'tʌmbl/ *v.* to fall down quickly and suddenly, especially with a rolling movement 跌倒，摔倒
e.g. Babies tumble when they are learning to walk.

recuse /rɪ'kjuːz/ *v.* to remove (oneself) from participation to avoid a conflict of interest 要求撤换
e.g. The judge recused himself from the case because he knew a member of the family.

mitigation /ˌmɪtɪ'geɪʃn/ *n.* the action of reducing the severity, seriousness, or painfulness of something 减轻；缓解
e.g. The planning process should have addressed mitigation of damage to the environment.

New Words and Expressions

gait /geɪt/ *n.* a particular way of walking 步态，步法

e.g. Melanie walked with the slightly awkward gait of a very tall person.

to five hours a night. I have a stiff gait usually when I begin walking after sitting for a while, loss of balance to some degree, losing common words or friends' names on occasion, a general forgetfulness…where's my phone, the car keys?

❻ I have put aside my goal of skiing when I turn 100. Otherwise my life hasn't changed much…that I've observed; which leads me to the title of my story…when will things begin deteriorating at an increased rate? What is next? Will I find I'm less tolerant of the next level of medications? When will I no longer be able to do those things I'm passionate about? I rarely think about these things mainly because I believe that I have no control over the progression of the disease and my neurologist and I will face each situation as they arise. So I enjoy the present and make future plans based on how I'm presently doing. Most importantly, I thank each day I have, days that I can share with my wife, kids, grand kids, and friends.

(647 words)

(Source: Ricky. 2020. Waiting for the Other Shoe to Drop. 11–23. From Parkinsons Disease website.)

Task

Text B has six paragraphs. Choose the correct summary for each of them from the list below.

List of Paragraph Summaries

1.	The medicine has almost no side effects for me, and I still lead a normal life.
2.	I cherish my present life since I don't know when my physical condition will become worse.
3.	My physical condition is quite normal, at the maximum dosage allowable, except for loss of balance as well as the left hand and foot shaking.
4.	It was three years later that I was diagnosed as early stage of Parkinson's disease, since the first noticed sign of left hand shaking.
5.	My Parkinson's disease might have begun earlier than 2015.
6.	I became a ski patroller after retirement from the army, for I cherished the opportunity to make the most of my physical skill.

Para. 1		Para. 2		Para. 3		Para. 4		Para. 5	

Para. 6	

Post-reading

Living with Bell's Palsy

New Words and Expressions

palsy /'pɔːlzɪ/ *n.* a loss of feeling in part of your body 瘫痪；麻痹；中风
e.g. Many children suffering from the cerebral palsy in China have been treated well.

droop /druːp/ *v.* to bend, hang, or move downwards, especially because of being weak or tired（尤指因衰弱或疲劳）低垂，垂落，下垂；萎靡
e.g. She was so tired, and her eyelids were beginning to droop.

slur /slɜː/ *v.* to be unable to pronounce each word clearly, because of being drunk, ill, or sleepy（因醉酒、生病或困乏）发音不清
e.g. He repeated himself and slurred his words more than usual.

❶ On May 22, 2017, I woke up with, what I jokingly refer to as a "broken face". I would later find out that this was Bell's **palsy**.

❷ Bell's palsy is a type of facial paralysis that results in an inability to control the facial muscles on the affected side. It's a condition in which the muscles on one side of your face become weak or paralyzed. It's caused by some kind of injury to the seventh cranial nerve. This is also called the "facial nerve". The most noticeable sign is weakness and **drooping** on one side of your face. You'll find it hard to close your eye on that side or make facial expressions like smiling. Your face may even be completely paralyzed on that side. It's rare, but Bell's palsy can sometimes affect the nerves in both sides of your face.

❸ Here is the story of my diagnosis and recovery.

❹ Initially, I wasn't scared. I had visited my GP who had diagnosed my condition, prescribed medicine, and sent me on my way. I went into work, worried, but determined that I would just "shrug this off". As the hours went on, I started to really panic. My speech became **slurred**, more of my face became paralyzed, and I had trouble with my eye closing and constantly watering. I ended up taking a trip to A & E and a few hours in and an MRI scan later—I was sent home with eye drops and a suggestion to buy an eye patch!

Getting My Bell's Palsy Diagnosis

5 I am quite a positive person but the first few days after my diagnosis were the hardest days I have ever faced. I couldn't eat or drink easily, as half of my face was paralyzed. I was exhausted, in constant pain and felt really down about my condition and my future. Slowly, I came round to the realization that I had this condition, but that it shouldn't stop me from living my life as best as I could. So with that **epiphany**—I went out and faced the world and have never looked back! I also quickly learned to find humor in things and I think this was a really key part of my recovery.

6 I joined the disability charity United Response in November 2018. They were really supportive. My manager here is really good with me and understands my condition. They couldn't be nicer! I can honestly say they really value their staff's well-being.

My Bell's Palsy Recovery

7 It's been nearly two years, and I am thrilled to say that I am 95% recovered. I have developed **synkinesis** (the result of incorrect wiring of nerves after trauma), but I am able to manage this with physiotherapy. I had a hard journey for the first year, I wasn't able to fully close my eyelid for five months, and I had to tape it closed on a night. Drinking was a mission as I didn't have control over my mouth, so straws became

---

New Words and Expressions

epiphany /ɪˈpɪfənɪ/ *n.* a moment of sudden insight or understanding 顿悟
e.g. I had an epiphany recently.

synkinesis /ˈsɪŋkɪniːsɪs/ *n.* a neurological symptom in which a voluntary muscle movement causes the simultaneous involuntary contraction of other muscles 联动症
e.g. Facial synkinesis is caused by trauma to the facial nerve.

my best friend. The hardest thing for me to deal with was the fatigue and **lethargy**.

❽ So, why am I sharing my story? Facial palsy is so common in the UK, yet not a lot is known about the condition and symptoms that go hand in hand with the palsy. I am also strangely thankful to have this condition. Whilst there is no known specific cause, most medical professionals believe there is a link between stress and developing the condition.

Raising Awareness of Bell's Palsy

❾ Since my diagnosis, I have completely changed my lifestyle and outlook on life. I allow myself time to rest and relax and have also learned, in the words of Elsa, to "Let it Go!" My diagnosis also came the same day as the evil attack at the MEN Arena. I consider myself very lucky, as I understand more than ever that tomorrow is never promised. I want to raise awareness of my condition and to promote the need for people to look after themselves mentally and emotionally.

(674 words)

(Source: Green, A. 2019. "I Woke Up with a Broken Face": Living with Bell's Palsy. 03–01. From United Response website.)

Your reading time: _____ mins

Your reading rate: _____ words/min

Read the text as quickly as you can and then choose the best answer to each question.

1. What can be said of Bell's palsy according to the text?

   A. It is mostly caused by stress.

   B. It is mostly related to people's mental health condition.

   C. It can be permanently cured soon.

   D. It is a specific type of facial paralysis.

2. Which of the following statements is true according to the text?

   A. The author has been optimistic all the time while fighting Bell's palsy.

   B. Epiphany implies a change of attitudes.

   C. The sixth cranial nerve is also known as the facial nerve.

   D. Bell's palsy does not affect the function of facial muscles.

3. What is the most challenging thing for the author to cope with during her recovery?

   A. Using straws.   B. Smiling.

   C. Tiredness and lack of enthusiasm.   D. Closing eyes.

4. Which of the following statements would the author most probably agree with?

   A. Facial paralysis only occurs on one side of the face.

   B. The best way to cure Bell's palsy is physiotherapy.

   C. Patients with Bell's palsy will not get fatigued during the treatment.

   D. People should pay attention to their own psychological and emotional health condition.

5. By saying "tomorrow is never promised", the author suggests that _____.

   A. we should make a promise today

   B. every "today" should be cherished

   C. we should never put off what we can do today until tomorrow

   D. we should always keep promise

Your comprehension rate: _____ %

Additional Reading

Small Steps So Far

New Words and Expressions

fiancée /fɪˈɒnseɪ/ *n.* the woman whom a man is going to marry 未婚妻

e.g. It would be unfair to marry your fiancée without being honest with her.

disk /dɪsk/ *n.* a small piece of cartilage (namely strong body tissue that stretches) between the bones of your back 椎间盘

e.g. He's been off work with a slipped disk.

---

❶ Egan Sarojak describes himself as an active 29-year-old man. He said he was feeling blessed after recently getting engaged and he and his **fiancée** have a baby on the way.

❷ As a regular golf player, Sarojak didn't think much of the weakness and soreness he occasionally felt in his legs, shrugging it off as a golf injury. The Danbury man figured he must have slipped a **disk** in his back, until he suddenly lost control of his legs and fell to the floor getting out of bed one morning.

❸ Unable to stand or walk, Sarojak crawled back to his bed and threw himself onto the mattress. His fiancée and friends picked him up and drove him to Danbury Hospital for help.

❹ Sarojak didn't know it at the time, but the weakness and soreness in his legs were signs of his developing Guillain-Barré (Ghee-yan Bahray) Syndrome (格林巴利综合征)—a rare neurological disorder with no known cause causing the body's immune system to attack its nerves, according to the Mayo Clinic.

❺ The syndrome affects approximately "one or two people in every 100,000 each year", according to the National Organization for Rare Disorders (NORD). It induces muscle weakness that in more severe cases evolves into nerve damage and paralysis, according to the National Institute of Neurological Disorders and Stroke (NINDS).

6 Sarojak's arms and legs were completely paralyzed, leaving him unable to even pick up his phone. He recalls watching his fingers stiffly "curl up" and feeling a burning pain in his legs and feet. Still, months later, he is grateful that the **prognosis** is just a rare, paralyzing disorder that he can fully recover from. The diagnosis was a good thing to him, better than being diagnosed with multiple sclerosis (MS, 多发性硬化症), amyotrophic lateral sclerosis (ALS, 肌萎缩性脊髓侧索硬化症), or diabetes, which he originally feared it was.

7 Lisa Antous, Sarojak's mother, struggled watching her son become "helpless".

8 "It was very hard at first. This is somebody who wouldn't even want to take an aspirin and he had to have a **heparin** shot in his stomach every day, three times a day," she said. Antous—motivated by her son's optimism—stood by Sarojak's hospital bed, tending to his needs in any way she could.

9 Sarojak spent a month at Danbury Hospital receiving high-dose **immunoglobulin** therapy (IVIG)—intravenous injections of immunoglobulin proteins that help attack infecting organisms—until he was discharged to the Gaylord Rehabilitation Hospital for recovery.

New Words and Expressions

prognosis /prɒgˈnəʊsɪs/ *n.* an estimate of the future of someone or something, especially about whether a patient will recover from an illness （尤指对病人能否康复的）预后
e.g. The doctor's prognosis was that Laurence might walk within 12 months.

heparin /ˈhepərɪn/ *n.* a compound occurring in the liver and other tissues which inhibits blood clotting 肝素
e.g. Heparin is used in the early treatment of blood clots in the lungs.

immunoglobulin /ˌɪmjʊnəʊˈglɒbjʊlɪn/ *n.* a class of proteins produced in lymph tissue in vertebrates and that function as antibodies in the immune response 免疫球蛋白
e.g. In the latter case, the cost of rabies vaccine and immunoglobulin alone exceeded $1,000,000.

New Words and Expressions

chip in to give some money, especially when several people are giving money to pay for something together 凑钱

e.g. They each chipped in $50 to take their parents out to dinner.

⑩ Community members are now supporting Sarojak through an uphill battle against a sudden and rare disorder.

⑪ "I couldn't believe what was going on; it was extremely overwhelming," Sarojak said of the support.

⑫ Sarojak was moved when he saw friends, community members, and strangers banding together to create a GoFundMe for his family that has since raised over $27,000. William Asmar—Sarojak's childhood friend—organized the donation to help his family cover remaining costs for his care and soon-to-be-born son.

⑬ "I think we all were happy to kind of **chip in** and make sure we could do what we can," Asmar said.

⑭ Sarojak's recovery time remains surrounded by question marks. Although some GBS patients recover in weeks, it can take years for others. "It's been three and a half months and it feels like it's been a year," Sarojak said.

⑮ He is experiencing small improvements in his arms and hands though his legs remain heavily unresponsive.

⑯ "We take the little victories that we get," Antous said.

⑰ He was given permission to go home but attends physical and occupational therapy sessions daily to reteach his nerves how to respond to messages from his brain.

⑱ In the last three months, Sarojak can only recount having five bad days. He feels overwhelming positivity and support from his family and the Greater Danbury Community that has put its arms around them.

⑲ He is learning basic functions **from scratch**. Learning how to hold a fork or walk again is just the beginning for Sarojak. "It's small steps so far...we're definitely going to get through it, and we have more support than we can possibly imagine," Sarojak said.

(668 words)

(Source: Colon, S. 2021. It's Small Steps So Far. 01–10. From Newstimes website.)

> **New Words and Expressions**
>
> **from scratch** from the beginning 从零开始
> **e.g.** Building a home from scratch can be both exciting and challenging.

Task

Read the text carefully and then complete the statements with appropriate words.

1. If you eat soon after your workout, you can minimize muscle stiffness and _____, and help reduce your fatigue.
2. Epilepsy is a chronic _____ disorder that affects people of all ages.
3. Most patients want to know even bad _____, but how much a physician tells a given patient should be determined primarily by the patient, not the physician.
4. He _____ the story of the interview for his first job.
5. It is generally accepted that people are _____ by success.
6. Physical _____ is an important aid to drug treatments.
7. Once on the scene, the police found Lewis lying _____ inside the home.
8. When we experience a quality issue, every team member should be willing to _____ to address the issue.

9. They still fill my life with _____, sincerity, and joy and inspire me to be more creative and productive.

10. Jack Ma established Alibaba, one of the most famous IT companies in China, from _____.

Unit **3** The Endocrine System

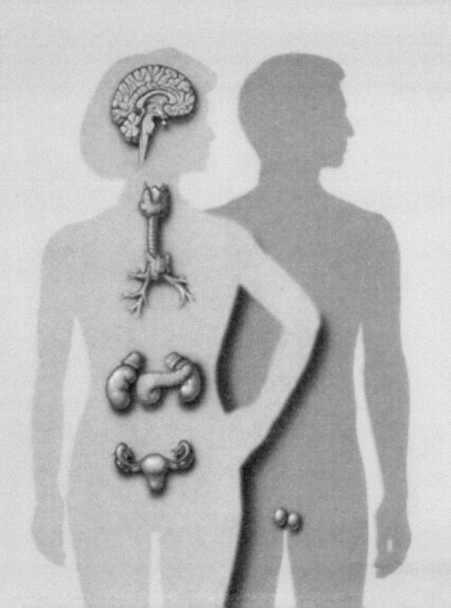

Pre-reading

The endocrine system is composed of glands and their chemical messengers called hormones. The endocrine system is instrumental in regulating growth and development, tissue function, metabolism, and reproductive processes. Hormones affect nearly every cell in the body by traveling through the bloodstream and binding to specialized receptors.

This unit firstly reviews the mysteries of some major endocrine glands and the most important hormones. Then, it briefly discusses the role of the endocrine system in growth and stress. Lastly, it reviews disorders of the endocrine system most relevant to human beings. You will be impressed by the functionality and complicacy of the endocrine system.

What are thyroid nodules? What is the truth about the human growth hormone (HGH) for weight loss? Do you know how to keep metabolism up and how to balance hormones? Read the following passages and see if you can find answers to these questions.

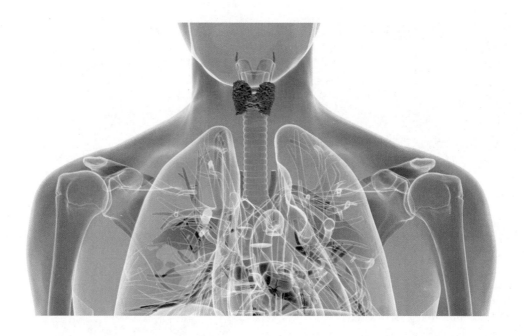

In-reading

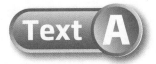

Thyroid Nodules

❶ **Thyroid nodules** are solid or fluid-filled lumps or bumps. They're found on your thyroid, a small, powerful **gland** in your neck. This gland makes thyroid hormones, which affect your metabolism (the internal process that turns your food into energy), heart rate, and many other systems in the body. Sometimes, cells in your thyroid can grow out of control and form a lump.

Are Thyroid Nodules Serious?

❷ Most often the answer is no. You usually can't feel thyroid nodules. Even though they happen from an overgrowth of cells, most thyroid nodules aren't cancer. About 1 in 10 thyroid nodules turn out to be cancer. Benign (non-cancerous) thyroid nodules are common. Lots of people get them as they get older. If a thyroid nodule isn't cancerous, it may not need any treatment. Doctors might just watch to make sure it doesn't keep growing or begin to cause other problems.

New Words and Expressions

thyroid /ˈθaɪrɔɪd/ *n.* an organ located near the base of the neck 甲状腺
e.g. The thyroid gland requires iodine to make the thyroid hormone.

nodule /ˈnɒdjuːl/ *n.* a small round lump or swelling 小结；小瘤；节结
e.g. On a complete physical exam, she notices a small thyroid nodule.

gland /ɡlænd/ *n.* an organ of the body which produces a substance that the body needs such as hormones, sweat, or saliva 腺
e.g. It is thought that being overweight may also increase the risk of cancer in the reproductive organs for women and in the prostate gland for men.

Types of Thyroid Nodules

❸   There are different types of thyroid nodules that aren't cancerous. Toxic nodules make too much thyroid hormone. This can lead to hyperthyroidism (甲状腺功能亢进), which makes the metabolism speed up. Multinodular goiters (甲状腺肿) have several nodules. They may also make too much thyroid hormone and may press on other structures. Thyroid cysts are full of fluid, sometimes with other debris. They may happen after an injury.

Symptoms of Thyroid Nodules

❹   Thyroid nodules usually don't have symptoms. If they are large, they may cause trouble breathing, trouble swallowing, a throat "tickle", and harshness or voice change. When a nodule causes the thyroid to make too much hormone, this is sometimes called a "hot nodule". It may cause weight loss, muscle weakness, heat intolerance, anxiousness, irritability, irregular heartbeat, and weak bones. Sometimes, people with thyroid nodules make too little thyroid hormone. This can cause symptoms of hypothyroidism (甲状腺功能减退): fatigue, cold sensitivity, constipation, dry skin, weight gain, **puffy** face, harshness, muscle weakness, high cholesterol, muscle aches, joint pain, thinning hair, depression, and memory loss.

Causes of Thyroid Nodules

❺   It's not always clear why a person gets thyroid nodules. Several medical conditions can cause them to form. **Thyroiditis**: This is chronic inflammation of the thyroid. One type of thyroiditis is called Hashimoto's disease (桥本氏病). It's associated with low thyroid activity (hypothyroidism). Iodine (碘) deficiency: A diet that lacks iodine can result in thyroid nodules. This is uncommon in the US, since iodine is added to many foods. Thyroid **adenoma**: This is an unexplained overgrowth of thyroid tissue. Most adenomas are harmless, but some produce thyroid hormones. This leads to an overactive thyroid (hyperthyroidism). Thyroid cancer: Most thyroid nodules aren't cancer, but some can be.

Diagnosing Thyroid Nodules

6 You may be able to identify one just by looking in the mirror. Face the mirror with your chin raised a little. Swallow and look for a bump on either side of your **windpipe** near your Adam's apple. Put your fingers gently on your neck in that spot and feel for a bump. If you find one, ask your doctor about it. About 90% of thyroid nodules are benign. If you notice one, have your doctor check it. For problems with your thyroid, you may want to see a specialist called an endocrinologist. Endocrinologists specialize in health problems related to the glands that make hormones, including the thyroid. They will do a physical exam and might order some tests to find out whether it's cancer or not. With a biopsy, your doctor will insert a very fine needle into your thyroid nodule to collect a few cells. They'll send them to a lab for further study. Non-cancerous thyroid nodules

> ## New Words and Expressions
>
> **adenoma** /ˌædɪˈnəʊmə/ *n.* a benign tumor of a glandular structure or of glandular origin 腺瘤
> **e.g.** The cut surface of the liver reveals the adenoma.
>
> **windpipe** /ˈwɪndpaɪp/ *n.* the main trunk of the system of tubes by which air passes to and from the lungs in vertebrates 气管；嗓门
> **e.g.** She gasps as if she's been punched in the windpipe.

can still be a problem if they grow too large and make it hard for you to breathe or swallow.

Treatment for Thyroid Nodules

7 When a nodule is not cancerous, treatment may include "watchful waiting" and thyroid hormone therapy. When nodules cause hyperthyroidism, treatment may include radioactive iodine, antithyroid medicines, beta blockers (β-受体阻滞药), and surgery. Any cancerous thyroid nodules should be removed surgically. The same is true for very large ones and those that change and develop strange features over time.

(667 words)

(Source: Nazario, B. 2020. Thyroid Nodules. 06–18. From Webmd website.)

Task One

Decide whether the following statements are true (T) or false (F) according to the text.

1. _____ Thyroid nodules have little to do with one's heart rate.

2. _____ People of all ages don't have equal odds to get thyroid nodules.

3. _____ Neither benign nor cancerous thyroid nodules usually have symptoms.

4. _____ Thyroid nodules cannot be identified by the naked eye.

5. _____ Non-cancerous thyroid nodules won't be a problem if they grow too large.

Task Two

Fill in the blanks with the words given below. Change their forms if necessary.

metabolism	gland	benign	toxic	hormone
constipation	inflammation	iodine	specialize	biopsy

1. In many places, like Japan, people get _____ from seafood, seaweed, and vegetables.
2. A college education will enable her to _____ in a certain field of knowledge.
3. James had a(n) _____ of the tumors over his right ear.
4. The sweating rate depends on the sweat output per _____.
5. Warm prune juice itself has been long used as a natural _____ remedy as well.
6. Too much _____ waste is being dumped into sea.
7. Chronic _____ is, of course, associated with major illnesses like heart disease and cancers.
8. The body's _____ is slowed down by extreme cold.
9. It wasn't cancer, only a(n) _____ tumor.
10. When the stem dies, its _____ signal also ceases.

Task Three

Paraphrase the following sentences from Text A.

1. This can lead to hyperthyroidism, which makes the metabolism speed up. (Para. 3)

   _____

   _____

   _____

   _____

2. They may also make too much thyroid hormone and may press on other structures. (Para. 3)

3. This is an unexplained overgrowth of thyroid tissue. (Para. 5)

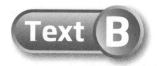

The Truth About HGH for Weight Loss

New Words and Expressions

pituitary gland /pɪˈtjuːɪtrɪ glænd/ a small organ at the base of the brain that controls the growth and activity of the body by producing hormones 脑下垂体

e.g. Hormone secretion is controlled by the pituitary gland.

❶ Can a naturally occurring hormone that promotes growth and development make a dieter's dream come true? The quest for an easier weight loss solution has some people taking HGH in pills, powders, and injections. A few small studies have linked HGH injections with fat loss and muscle gain. But the changes seen were minimal—just a few pounds—while the risks and potential side effects are not.

How HGH Works?

❷ HGH is produced by the **pituitary gland**

to fuel growth and development in children. It also maintains some bodily functions, like tissue repair, muscle growth, brain function, energy, and metabolism, throughout life.

❸ HGH production peaks during the teenage years and slowly declines with age. Studies have shown that obese adults have lower levels than normal-weight adults. And these lower levels of HGH have some people wondering whether a boost of HGH could enhance weight loss, especially in the obese. HGH has also gained a reputation as a muscle builder, and its use is banned in the Olympics and other sports. However, there is little solid evidence that it can boost athletic performance.

Early Study Sparks Interest in HGH

❹ Interest in using HGH for weight loss stems from a study in *New England Journal of Medicine* in 1990 that showed injections of synthetic HGH resulted in 8.8% gain in muscle mass and 14% loss in body fat without any change in diet or exercise. Although this study appeared to be promising, many later studies have shown no such benefit. In March 2003, the same journal took the unusual step of **denouncing** misuse of the study in 1990, pointing out that subsequent reports provided no reason to be optimistic. Despite this, the study in 1990 is still being used to promote Internet sales of HGH for weight loss.

Small Changes, But No Weight Loss

❺ When adults with an HGH deficiency resulting from pituitary disease are given HGH

New Words and Expressions

denounce /dɪˈnaʊns/ *v.* to criticize something or someone strongly and publicly 谴责

e.g. We must denounce injustice and oppression.

replacement, it improves **body composition**—increasing bone mass and muscle mass and decreasing fat stores. But it does not cause weight loss in the obese, says Nicholas Tritos, MD, who co-authored an analysis evaluating the effectiveness of HGH for weight loss in obese people. "Our results showed small improvements in body composition, a small reduction in body fat and increase in muscle mass, but on balance, weight did not change," he says. "More notable changes are seen when an individual is deficient in the growth hormone from true pituitary disease." Another study found that HGH therapy was linked to a small decrease in fat and increase in lean mass, but no change in body weight. The researchers concluded that HGH is not an effective treatment in obese people, and more studies were needed.

Pills and Powders: Risky and Expensive

❻ HGH comes in the injectable form, usually given once weekly, and is available only with a doctor's prescription. HGH injections are approved to treat adults and children who have growth hormone deficiency, for people who are undergoing organ transplants, and for AIDS-related muscle wasting. Companies marketing HGH pills and powders claim their products produce the same effects as the injected form. But Tritos warns that HGH is only effective when injected.

❼ The FDA has not approved HGH for weight loss for a variety of reasons, including the cost, potential **aggravation** of insulin resistance and other side effects, and lack of long-term safety studies. Healthy adults who take HGH put themselves at risk for joint and muscle pain, swelling in the arms and legs, carpel tunnel syndrome (腕管综合征), and insulin resistance. In the elderly, these symptoms are more profound.

The Bottom Line

8   Using HGH for weight loss, muscle building, or anti-aging is experimental and **controversial**. HGH injections are believed to decrease fat storage and increase muscle growth to some extent, but studies have not shown this to be a safe or effective weight loss remedy. Until more research can demonstrate the long-term safety and effectiveness of using HGH for weight loss, it's wise to avoid it. Unfortunately, there are no magic bullets when it comes to losing weight. Healthy weight loss means taking in fewer calories than you burn in physical activity. Save your money for more fruits and vegetables, and a good pair of **sneakers**.

New Words and Expressions

controversial /ˌkɒntrəˈvɜːʃl/ *adj.* causing disagreement or discussion 有争议的；有争论的
e.g. The book was very controversial.

sneaker /ˈsniːkə/ *n.* a casual shoe with a rubber sole that people wear often for running or other sports 运动鞋
e.g. He wore old jeans and a pair of sneakers.

(698 words)

(Source: Danko, I. 2020. The Truth About HGH for Weight Loss. 05–24. From Ivandanko website.)

Text B has eight paragraphs. Choose the correct summary for each of them from the list below.

List of Paragraph Summaries

1.	HGH brings changes, but no weight loss.
2.	HGH injections are approved to treat patients.
3.	Weight loss by pills is no longer a dream but remains to be risky.
4.	HGH has potential side effects, so it's not approved by the FDA for weight loss.
5.	HGH is produced to help with the growth of children and some bodily functions.
6.	It's wise to avoid using HGH for weight loss, because it's experimental and controversial.
7.	Whether a boost of HGH could enhance weight loss or athlete performance is unknown.
8.	The study in 1990 sparked interest in using HGH for weight loss, but subsequent reports provide no reason to be optimistic.

Para. 1		Para. 2		Para. 3		Para. 4		Para. 5	
Para. 6		Para. 7		Para. 8					

Post-reading

How to Maintain Your Metabolism

❶ Do you find that, lately, you get full more quickly or your weight has started creeping up and you're not sure why? A drop in your metabolism may be to blame.

❷ Metabolism is the rate at which your body uses energy or burns calories, and it's dependent on a variety of factors. "It takes a certain amount of energy just to breathe, but your metabolism also includes your daily activities and all the chemical reactions going on in your body—everything from breaking down food to building cellular structures," says Reyhan Westbrook, PhD, an instructor of **geriatrics** and **gerontology** at the Johns Hopkins School of Medicine in Baltimore.

❸ Here are three factors that can slow your metabolism—and the steps you can take to keep it going strong. "The main reasons for the decline of metabolism are biological, but your lifestyle also plays a major role," says Zhaoping Li, MD, PhD, a professor of medicine and director of the UCLA Center for Human Nutrition at the David Geffen School of Medicine.

Reasons Why the Calorie Burn Slows

❹ **Age:** Muscle is a major calorie burner. But after age 30, muscle mass decreases approximately

New Words and Expressions

geriatrics /ˌdʒerɪˈætrɪks/ *n.* the study of the illnesses that affect old people and the medical care of old people 老年病学

e.g. An old family member is often the inspiration for medical students who choose geriatrics.

gerontology /ˌdʒerɒnˈtɒlədʒɪ/ *n.* the comprehensive multidisciplinary study of aging and older adults 老年医学；老年病学；老年学

e.g. I have decided to study gerontology at college.

3% to 8% per decade. Because muscle burns more calories than fat, that decline can significantly reduce the amount of energy your body needs. "People also tend to be less active as they age, which decreases their energy (calorie) output," Westbrook says. But changes in muscle mass and physical activity are only part of the **equation**. Activity inside of your body's cells also slows down with age.

❺ **Mental health:** Anxiety can also put the brakes on your metabolism. A study in 2015 published in the journal *Biological Psychiatry* found that stress causes a decrease in calorie burning following a high-fat meal. "Since people tend to eat high-fat meals when they're stressed, this could be a common occurrence," says Janice Kiecolt-Glaser, PhD, the director of the Institute for Behavioral Medicine Research at Ohio State University College of Medicine and the study's lead researcher. Experts also suspect a link between depression and metabolism. "Depression has a direct impact on your appetite, food choices, and activity level," Li says.

❻ **Sleep:** "Getting enough sleep, going to bed, and waking up at consistent times, may help you burn fat more efficiently," Westbrook says. The National Sleep Foundation recommends that older adults get seven to eight hours of sleep per night, but health problems and medications often get in the way.

Keeping Your Metabolism Up

⑦   When faced with a slowing metabolism, your first instinct may be to eat less, but that can **backfire**. "When you restrict calories, you run the risk of not taking in enough protein, which can result in more muscle loss," Li says.

⑧   Even if you find that you get full more easily than you once did, it's important to make sure you're getting the nutrients you need.

⑨   Focus on eating enough protein (the building block of muscle). The dietary reference intake is 0.8 gram per kilogram of body weight (about 51 grams for a 140-pound person), but experts suggest that people aged 55 and older get a bit more. "Aim for at least 20 grams of protein per meal, or make 20% to 25% of every meal protein," Li says. Try to include the nutrient every time you eat, rather than having all your protein in one sitting. Along with meat and seafood, eggs, cheese, nuts, and beans, all provide ample amounts of protein.

⑩   Building and preserving your muscle mass through strength training can also help keep your metabolism up. "Exercise like running and swimming promotes heart health, but resistance exercise preserves muscle mass," Westbrook says. And research shows that your resting metabolic rate stays elevated by about 5% to 7% for up to 72 hours after a resistance session.

⑪   And don't forget the importance of mental health and sleep. If you're feeling **persistent**

New Words and Expressions

backfire /ˌbækˈfaɪə/ *v.* to come back to the originator of an action with an undesired effect 产生出乎意料及事与愿违的结果
e.g. While this may seem justified by a noble goal, such "policy by people" tactics rarely work and often backfire.

persistent /pəˈsɪstənt/ *adj.* existing for a long or longer than usual time or continuously 持续的；持久的
e.g. I had a persistent cough for over a month.

sadness or stress, talk to your doctor; to improve your sleep, exercise daily, stick to a consistent bedtime, and avoid alcohol and caffeine before bed.

(669 words)

(Source: Detz, J. 2020. How to Maintain Your Metabolism. 02–24. From Consumer Reports website.)

Your reading time: _____ mins

Your reading rate: _____ words/min

Task

Read the text as quickly as you can and then choose the best answer to each question.

1. Metabolism is the rate at which your body _____.

 A. uses energy or burns calories   B. absorbs energy

 C. absorbs and uses energy   D. generates hormones

2. Metabolism does not include _____.

 A. your daily activities

 B. all the chemical reactions going on in your body

 C. building cellular structures

 D. diarrhea and constipation

3. The main reasons for the decline of metabolism are as follows except the _____.

 A. mental health   B. lifestyle

 C. aging   D. gene

4. Which of the following is not the right way to keep metabolism up?

 A. Eating enough protein.   B. Strengthening the body.

C. Keeping a 6-hour sleep per day.   D. Having a light mood.

5. Which of the following statements is true according to the text?

A. Having little meat is good for metabolism.

B. Sleeping longer than eight hours a day slows down your metabolism.

C. Stress can help burn the calories.

D. Restricting calories is risky of not taking in enough protein.

Your comprehension rate: _____ %

Additional Reading

Natural Ways to Balance Your Hormones

❶   Hormones have profound effects on your mental, physical, and emotional health. These chemical messengers play a major role in controlling your appetite, weight, and mood, among other things. Normally, your endocrine glands produce the precise amount of each hormone needed for various processes in your body. However, hormonal imbalances have become increasingly common with today's fast-paced modern lifestyle. In addition, certain hormones decline with age, and some people experience a more **dramatic** decrease than others. Fortunately, a nutritious diet and other healthy lifestyle behaviors may help improve your hormonal health and allow you to feel and

New Words and Expressions

dramatic /drə'mætɪk/ *adj.* very sudden or noticeable, or full of action and excitement 巨大的；剧烈的
e.g. There has been a dramatic shift in public opinion towards peaceful negotiations.

New Words and Expressions

ghrelin /'grelɪn/ *n.* a hormone produced in the body that stimulates appetite 饥饿激素

e.g. When ghrelin levels are up, people feel hungry.

perform your best. The text will show you two natural ways to balance your hormones.

Eat Enough Protein at Every Meal

❷ Consuming an adequate amount of protein is extremely important. Dietary protein provides essential amino acids (氨基酸) that your body can't make on its own and must be consumed every day in order to maintain muscle, bone, and skin health. In addition, protein influences the release of hormones that control appetite and food intake.

❸ Research has shown that eating protein decreases levels of the "hunger hormone" **ghrelin** and stimulates the production of hormones that help you feel full, including PYY and GLP-1.

❹ In one study, men produced 20% more GLP-1 and 14% more PYY after eating a high-protein meal than after eating a meal that contained a normal amount of protein. What's more, participants' hunger ratings decreased by 25% more after the high-protein meal compared to the normal-protein meal. In another study, women who consumed a diet containing 30% protein experienced an increase in GLP-1 and greater feelings of fullness than when they ate a diet containing 10% protein. What's more, they experienced an increase in metabolism and fat burning.

❺ To optimize hormone health, experts recommend consuming a minimum of 20–30 grams of protein per meal. This is easy to do by including a serving of these high-protein foods at each meal.

6 Consuming adequate protein triggers the production of hormones that suppress appetite and help you feel full. Aim for a minimum of 20–30 grams of protein per meal.

Engage in Regular Exercise

7 Physical activity can strongly influence hormonal health. A major benefit of exercise is its ability to reduce insulin levels and increase insulin sensitivity.

8 Insulin is a hormone that has several functions. One is allowing cells to take up sugar and amino acids from the bloodstream, which are then used for energy and maintaining muscle. However, a little insulin goes a long way. Too much can be **downright** dangerous. High insulin levels have been linked to inflammation, heart disease, diabetes, and cancer. What's more, they are connected to insulin resistance, a condition in which your cells don't respond properly to insulin's signals.

9 Many types of physical activity have been found to increase insulin sensitivity and reduce insulin levels, including adiponectin (脂联素) exercise, strength training, and endurance exercise. In a 24-week study of obese women, exercise increased participants' insulin sensitivity and levels of adiponectin, a hormone that has anti-inflammatory effects and helps regulate metabolism. Being physically active may also help boost levels of muscle-maintaining hormones that decline with age such as testosterone, IGF-1, DHEA, and growth hormones.

New Words and Expressions

downright /ˈdaʊnraɪt/ *adv.* absolutely（强调令人不快或负面的事或行为）彻头彻尾地；十足地；完全地
e.g. "Thanks" can be useful, as it is able to bridge the divide between the formality of "thank you" and the downright relaxed "cheers".

❿ For people who are unable to perform **vigorous** exercise, even regular walking may increase these hormone levels, potentially improving strength and quality of life. Although a combination of resistance and aerobic training seems to provide the best results, engaging in any type of physical activity on a regular basis is beneficial.

⓫ Performing strength training, aerobics, walking, or other forms of physical activity can modify hormone levels in a way that reduces the risk of disease and protects muscle mass during the aging process.

(607 words)

(Source: Smith, L. 2020. Natural Ways to Balance Your Hormones. 01–29. From Keep Women Healthy website.)

Task

Read the text and complete the statements with appropriate words.

1. To learn more about the _____ system, watch this ADAM animation.
2. _____ exercise gets the heart pumping and helps you burn fat.
3. Blindness is a common complication of _____.
4. _____ is secreted by the pancreas.
5. Junk foods are anything but _____, so students should avoid them.
6. _____ acids are the building blocks of proteins.
7. The man was _____ rude to us.
8. Very _____ exercise can increase the risk of heart attacks.
9. They want all groups to be treated on an equal _____.
10. Drug traffickers continue to flourish despite international attempts to _____ them.

Unit 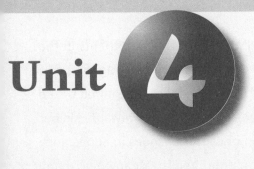 4 The Integumentary System

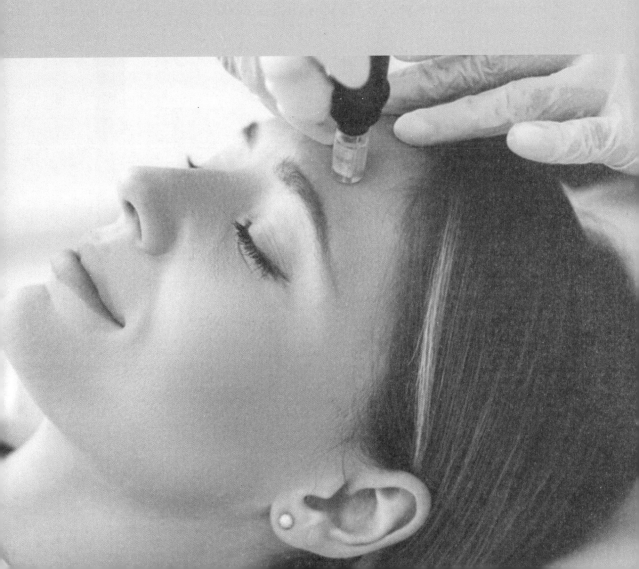

Pre-reading

The skin, a mirror of human health, keeps vital chemicals and nutrients in the body while providing a barrier against dangerous substances from entering the body. It also provides a shield from the harmful effects of ultraviolet radiation emitted by the sun. Smooth, healthy, and vibrant skin is appreciated, sought after, and rewarded in our society. Anything that interferes with skin function or causes changes in appearance can have major consequences for physical and mental health. Meanwhile, many problems that appear on the skin provide clues to a disorder that affects the entire body.

What causes the inevitable skin aging? What can be done to protect our skin while we are enjoying a wonderful and pleasant sunbath? Do we need special skin care during the coronavirus pandemic and why? This unit will throw light on skin aging and skin problems and offer you a better access to healthy skin.

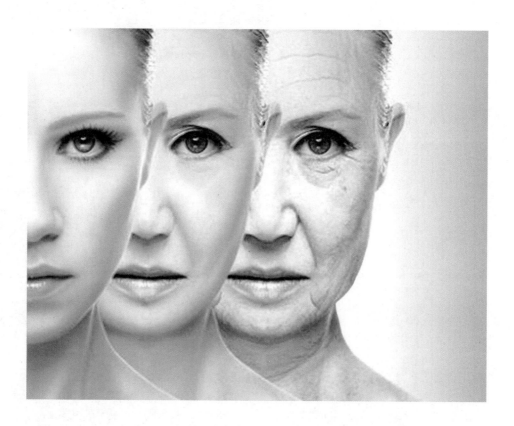

In-reading

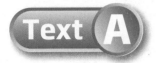

The Factors of Skin Aging

❶ Skin aging is divided into two categories—intrinsic and extrinsic. Intrinsic aging comprises age-related changes that are not under your control, like genetic factors. Extrinsic aging includes factors that you actually can control, like exposure to sun. Here is a brief but very beneficial overview of these factors that will give you important clues to what you can do today to keep your skin young longer.

Key Factors of Intrinsic Aging

❷ **Heredity:** Your genetic factors **dictate** the rate at which your aging process progresses. Paying attention to how your parents' skin was aging can be very useful. If one or both of your parents had youthful skin well into the old age, chances are that you could inherit the same characteristics.

❸ **Hormones:** The most dramatic changes in women's appearance take place around menopause years, when **estrogen** drop causes considerable loss of collagen (胶原), which is

> ### New Words and Expressions
>
> **dictate** /dɪk'teɪt/ *v.* to control or influence something 决定；支配；影响
> **e.g.** Of course, a number of factors will dictate how long an apple tree can survive.
>
> **estrogen** /'iːstrədʒn/ *n.* a general term for female steroid sex hormones that are secreted by the ovary and responsible for typical female sexual characteristics 雌激素
> **e.g.** The estrogen in birth control pills may increase blood coagulation.

an important protein that makes up most of the skin's supportive structure. As a result, wrinkles appear and skin hangs loosely.

❹ **Cellular recession:** The process of aging originates at the microscopic level, i.e. at the level of each individual cell. When the numerous functions at the cellular level are impaired, the cell cannot perform the metabolic and regenerating activities that promote health of the skin. This results in such visible signs of aging as wrinkles, skin sagging, and furrows.

Key Factors of Extrinsic Aging

❺ Fortunately the factors that have the biggest impact on your skin aging are extrinsic, i.e. you can control them to enhance the look of your skin and keep it young for longer.

❻ **Sun exposure:** There is no single factor of premature skin aging that has greater influence than sunlight. According to estimation of researchers, damage caused by ultraviolet rays of the sun is responsible for up to 80% of skin aging.

❼ The main reason why the sunlight is so harmful to the skin is that it triggers the production of free radicals (自由基) in the skin. A free radical is an atom or molecule that bears an unpaired electron and is extremely reactive, capable of engaging in rapid chain reactions that **destabilize** other molecules and generate many more free radicals.

❽ Excess of free radicals is related to increased risk of many chronic diseases, including cancer and stroke. When produced in skin, free radicals attack its collagen. As a result, skin loses its resilience and develops wrinkles.

❾ Most of the sun damage happens in the early part of our lives, when our cheeks are still glowing with freshness of youth, but the results do not appear until we are in our late 30s or 40s.

❿ Smoking: "Smoker's face" is a term used by doctors to describe the characteristic changes that happen to the faces of many people who smoke. The general appearance is of accelerated aging of the face, with a characteristic pattern of facial wrinkling and **sallow** coloration.

⓫ Smoking decreases the flow of oxygen to the skin by as much as 30%. Fine blood vessels in the **dermis** of the skin narrow, which cuts off the supply of nutrients that are necessary for constant self-regeneration of the skin and removal of waste products. As a result, skin begins to look gray and dull.

⓬ Smoking also triggers the production of free radicals in the body. Besides upsetting balance of bodily tissues and organs, the free radicals attack collagen of the skin, making it lose its **elasticity** and resilience.

⓭ Wear and tear: It is also a factor of skin aging. These are expression lines that appear on your face when you smile or frown. Over time this leaves permanent stamp on your face due to constant mechanical challenge. It is pretty hard to avoid, but there is still something you can do about it.

New Words and Expressions

sallow /ˈsæləʊ/ *adj.* (of a person's skin) having a slightly yellow color that does not look healthy 蜡黄的；灰黄的
e.g. Her sallow skin was drawn tightly across the bones of her face.

dermis /ˈdɜːmɪs/ *n.* the deep vascular inner layer of the skin 真皮
e.g. We may say that the epidermis protects the dermis.

elasticity /ˌiːlæˈstɪsɪtɪ/ *n.* the ability to bounce 弹力；弹性
e.g. The skin eventually loses its elasticity.

⑭ Lifestyle habits: Such factors like your eating habits, how much sleep you get, the degree of stress to which you are exposed, the amount and type of exercise you engage also affect your skin.

⑮ Healthy habits slow progression of aging of your whole body as well as your skin. Introducing simple changes in your daily routine has a great potential for improving the condition of your skin.

(686 words)

(Source: Anon. 2020. The Factors of Skin Aging. 01–29. From Ask Women Net website.)

Task One

Decide whether the following statements are true (T) or false (F) according to the text.

1. _____ Skin aging caused by intrinsic or extrinsic factors can't be controlled.

2. _____ Genes from parents can somehow determine the rate of the aging process.

3. _____ Intrinsic factors are more important to affect your skin aging than extrinsic ones.

4. _____ Smoking can speed up skin aging mainly because it directly changes skin into yellow.

5. _____ Facial expressions like smiles or frowns can accelerate your skin aging.

Task Two

Fill in the blanks with the words and phrase given below. Change their forms if necessary.

comprise	beneficial	inherit	considerable	originate
enhance	premature	trigger	accelerate	wear and tear

1. In order to catch up with and surpass the advanced world levels, we'll have to _____ our speed.
2. We _____ from our parents many of our physical characteristics.
3. This hereditary unit _____ a single complementation group, or in other words a single gene.
4. Nowadays a(n) _____ baby has a very good chance of survival.
5. Mother's Day _____ in America during the early 20th century.
6. The illness is _____ by a chemical imbalance in the brain.
7. There is _____ disagreement over the safety of the treatment.
8. These products can stand _____.
9. A good diet is _____ to health.
10. The drug increases the number of red cells in the blood, _____ oxygen uptake by 10%.

Task Three

Paraphrase the following sentences from Text A.

1. Your genetic factors dictate the rate at which your aging process progresses. (Para. 2)

   _____

   _____

   _____

   _____

2. When the numerous functions at the cellular level are impaired, the cell cannot perform the metabolic and regenerating activities that promote health of the skin. (Para. 4)

_____

_____

_____

_____

3. Over time this leaves permanent stamp on your face due to constant mechanical challenge. (Para. 13)

_____

_____

_____

_____

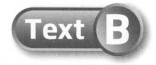

How to Treat Sunburn

❶　The sun, tanning lights, or any other source of ultraviolet light can cause sunburn or reddened, tender skin. Prevention is better than the cure, especially as the accompanying skin damage is permanent, but there are treatments available to encourage healing, prevent infection, and reduce pain.

Relieving Pain and Discomfort

② Keep the water just below lukewarm (cool, but not tooth-chattering cold) and relax for 10 to 20 minutes. If showering, use a gentle stream of water, not a full blast, to avoid irritating your skin. Air dry or pat gently with a towel to avoid **abrading** the skin. Avoid using soap, bath oils, or other **detergents** as you bathe or shower. Any such products can irritate your skin and possibly make the effects of the sunburn even worse. If you have blisters forming on your skin, take a bath instead of showering. The pressure from the shower might pop your blisters.

③ Dampen a washcloth or other piece of fabric with cold water, and lay it over the affected area for 20 to 30 minutes. Re-wet it as often as you need to.

④ Over-the-counter drugs such as aspirin can lessen the pain, and may or may not reduce inflammation. Do not give aspirin to children. Instead, opt for something that is specifically marketed as a child's dose of fever medicine.

⑤ Drugstores also sell sprays meant to relieve red and itchy skin. Sprays that contain **anesthetic** ingredients have a numbing effect that may help with the pain. However, as these are potential **allergens**, it may be best to test the medication on an unaffected patch of skin first and wait a day to see if it causes itchiness or redness. These sprays should not be used on children two years of age or younger without a doctor's advice.

⑥ Baggy T-shirts and loose cotton pajama

New Words and Expressions

abrade /əˈbreɪd/ *v.* to rub hard or scrub 磨损；擦伤
e.g. The cook is trying to abrade carrots into threads.

detergent /dɪˈtɜːdʒənt/ *n.* a chemical substance, usually in the form of a powder or liquid, which is used for washing things such as clothes or dishes 清洁剂；洗涤剂；去垢剂
e.g. No detergent can shift these stains.

anesthetic /ˌænəsˈθetɪk/ *n.* a drug that causes temporary loss of bodily sensations 麻醉药；麻醉剂
e.g. I cannot do a procedure like this without an anesthetic.

allergen /ˈælədʒən/ *n.* any substance that can cause an allergy 过敏原
e.g. When the immune system encounters an allergen, it may become sensitized.

pharmacist /ˈfɑːməsɪst/ *n.* a health professional trained in the art of preparing and dispensing drugs 药剂师
e.g. The pharmacist labeled the bottle poison.

pants are ideal clothing items to wear while you're recovering from sunburn. If you can't wear loose clothing, at least make sure your garments are cotton (this fabric allows your skin to "breathe") and fit as loosely as possible. Wool and some synthetic fabrics are especially irritating, due to scratchy fibers or trapped heat.

❼ Cortisone (皮质酮) cream contains steroidal (类固醇的) treatments that may reduce inflammation, although evidence suggests that they have little effect on sunburn. If you think it's worth a try, you can find low-dose, over-the-counter tubes at your local drugstore or supermarket. Look for hydrocortisone (氢羟肾上腺皮质素) or something similar. Do not use cortisone cream on young children, or in the face region. Ask your **pharmacist** for advice if you have any doubts or concerns about using this cream.

Preventing Re-exposure and Further Damage

❽ Ideally, you should hang out in the shade or wear clothing over affected areas if you're going back out into the sunshine.

❾ Use a sunscreen with at least SPF (防晒系数) 30 whenever you go outside. Reapply every hour, after exposure to water or excessive sweat, or according to the product label.

❿ Sunburn can be dehydrating, so it's important to counterbalance this by drinking plenty of water while you recover. Eight to ten glasses of water a day are recommended while recovering, with each glass containing one cup (240 mL) of water.

⑪ When you no longer have open blisters or the redness of the sunburn has subsided a bit, you can safely use a moisturizing cream. Liberally apply a creamy, unscented moisturizer to sunburned areas over the next few days or weeks to prevent peeling and irritation.

⑫ Contact a doctor immediately if your skin is blistering from sunburn. A sign of severe sunburn should be treated with personal medical advice, and the blisters put you at risk of infection. While waiting for an appointment, or if your doctor does not recommend any specific treatment, do remember to leave blisters intact or protect blisters with a clean dressing.

(628 words)

(Source: Lee, L. 2021. How to Treat a Sunburn. 04–18. From WikiHow website.)

Task

Text B has twelve paragraphs. Choose the correct summary for each of them from the list below (Paragraph one and twelve not included).

List of Paragraph Summaries

1.	Drink enough water.
2.	Consider cortisone creams.
3.	Try sprays to relieve pain.
4.	Wear a sunscreen.

5.	Use a cold, wet compress.
6.	Apply a moisturizer.
7.	Take a cool bath or gentle shower.
8.	Minimize sun exposure.
9.	Take a pain reliever.
10.	Wear loose cotton clothing over sunburned areas.

Para. 2		Para. 3		Para. 4		Para. 5		Para. 6	
Para. 7		Para. 8		Para. 9		Para. 10		Para. 11	

Post-reading

Skin Care: Five Tips for Healthy Skin

New Words and Expressions

pamper /ˈpæmpə/ v. to treat with excessive indulgence 善待；纵容；溺爱
e.g. Grandparents often pamper the children.

❶ Good skin care—including sun protection and gentle cleansing—can keep your skin healthy and glowing.

❷ You don't have time for intensive skin care? You can still **pamper** yourself by acing the basics. Good skin care and healthy lifestyle choices can help delay natural aging and prevent various skin problems. Get started with these five no-nonsense tips.

Protect Yourself from the Sun

③ One of the most important ways to take care of your skin is to protect it from the sun. A lifetime of sun exposure can cause wrinkles, age spots, and other skin problems—as well as increase the risk of skin cancer.

④ For the most complete sun protection:

- **Use a sunscreen.** Use a broad-spectrum sunscreen with an SPF of at least 15. Apply sunscreen generously, and reapply every two hours—or more often if you're swimming or perspiring.

- **Seek shade.** Avoid the sun between 10 am and 4 pm, when the sun's rays are the strongest.

- **Wear protective clothing.** Cover your skin with tightly woven long-sleeved shirts, long pants, and wide-brimmed hats. Also consider laundry additives, which give clothing an additional layer of ultraviolet protection for a certain number of washing, or special sun-protective clothing—which is specifically designed to block ultraviolet rays.

Don't Smoke

⑤ Smoking makes your skin look older and contributes to wrinkles. Smoking narrows the tiny blood vessels in the outermost layers of skin, which decreases blood flow and makes skin paler. This also **depletes** the skin of oxygen and nutrients that are important to skin health.

New Words and Expressions

deplete /dɪˈpliːt/ *v.* to lessen greatly in amount, contents, etc. 使大大地减少；使空虚
e.g. Mankind must take care not to deplete the earth of its natural resources.

❻ Smoking also damages collagen and **elastin**—the fibers that give your skin strength and elasticity. In addition, the repetitive facial expressions you make when smoking—such as pursing your lips when inhaling and squinting your eyes to keep out smoke—can contribute to wrinkles.

❼ In addition, smoking increases your risk of **squamous** cell skin cancer. If you smoke, the best way to protect your skin is to quit. Ask your doctor for tips or treatments to help you stop smoking.

Treat Your Skin Gently

❽ Daily cleansing and shaving can take a toll on your skin. To keep it gentle:

- **Limit bath time.** Hot water and long showers or baths remove oils from your skin. Limit your bath or shower time, and use warm—rather than hot—water.

- **Avoid strong soaps.** Strong soaps and detergents can strip oil from your skin. Instead, choose mild cleansers.

- **Shave carefully.** To protect and **lubricate** your skin, apply shaving cream, **lotion**, or gel before shaving. For the closest shave, use a clean, sharp razor. Shave in the direction the hair grows, not against it.

- **Pat your skin dry.** After washing or bathing, gently pat or blot your skin dry with a towel so that some moisture remains on your skin.

- **Moisturize dry skin.** If your skin is dry, use a moisturizer that fits your skin type. For daily use, consider a moisturizer that contains SPF.

Eat a Healthy Diet

9 A healthy diet can help you look and feel your best. Eat plenty of fruits, vegetables, whole grains, and lean proteins. The association between diet and acne isn't clear—but some research suggests that a diet rich in fish oil or fish oil supplements and low in unhealthy fats and processed or refined carbohydrates might promote younger looking skin. Drinking plenty of water helps keep your skin hydrated.

Manage Stress

10 Uncontrolled stress can make your skin more sensitive and trigger acne breakouts and other skin problems. To encourage healthy skin—and a healthy state of mind—take steps to manage your stress. Get enough sleep, set reasonable limits, **scale back** your to-do list, and make time to do the things you enjoy. The results might be more dramatic than you expect.

(617 words)

(Source: Anon. 2019. Skin Care: 5 Tips for Healthy Skin. 10–15. From Mayo Clinic website.)

New Words and Expressions

scale back to reduce something, especially an amount of money or business, etc. 削减；裁减

e.g. Despite current price advantage, UK manufacturers are still having to scale back production.

Your reading time: _____ mins

Your reading rate: _____ words/min

Read the text as quickly as you can and then choose the best answer to each question.

1. What can help delay natural aging according to the text?

    A. Taking a bath a little longer than usual every day.

    B. Drinking a lot of water every day.

    C. Sleeping as much as one can each day.

    D. Good skin care and a healthy lifestyle.

2. Which of the following statements is true?

    A. If we don't have time for intensive skin care, we can do nothing for our skin.

    B. Smoking can decrease blood flow and make skin paler.

    C. It is unnecessary to apply a sunscreen while we are swimming.

    D. Stress can cause skin problems in any case.

3. Smoking can cause skin problems in that _____.

    A. smoking narrows the tiny blood vessels in the outermost layers of skin, which decreases blood flow

    B. smoking damages the fibers that give your skin strength and elasticity

    C. smoking increases your risk of squamous cell skin cancer

    D. All of the above.

4. To treat our skin correctly and gently, we should _____.

    A. moisturize dry skin with a moisturizer that fits our skin type

    B. bath and shave with hot water every day

    C. clean our skin with strong soaps and detergents

    D. keep our skin dry quickly with a towel

5. Which of the following is not the way to manage our stress according to the text?

    A. To get enough sleep.

    B. To set reasonable limits.

    C. To reduce appropriately your to-do list and make time to do the things you enjoy.

    D. To do more exercises.

Your comprehension rate: _____ %

Additional Reading

Upgrading Your Skincare Routine During the Coronavirus Pandemic

❶　From the very start of the coronavirus pandemic, the recommendation to wash your hands more often—and the correct way—was rightfully **touted** as one of the most important methods for preventing virus transmission.

❷　Keeping your skin moisturized is an important step in preventing coronavirus, since germs can get into cracked, dry skin, but there's a crucial next step that hasn't received as much attention: keeping your skin moisturized to prevent the kind of cracking and micro-tears that could make you more susceptible to COVID-19. If you don't rehydrate, ironically, washing your hands frequently could, indirectly, be putting you at higher risk.

❸　Another potential risk factor is the dry skin you may experience from wearing face masks, which makes it tougher to adhere to the other recommendation: "Don't touch your face."

❹　Why dry skin is a problem? Frequent washing can cause a loss of natural oils—called **sebum**—on the skin, but sebum helps maintain the skin's healthy barrier which protects you from the outside world. Especially for runners who are still logging miles (safely and alone!)

New Words and Expressions

tout /taʊt/ *v.* to advertise in strongly positive terms 吹捧；兜售
e.g. The politician was touted as a friend of people.

sebum /ˈsiːbəm/ *n.* an oily substance produced by glands in the skin 皮脂
e.g. The sebum travels through these passages.

New Words and Expressions

erratic /ɪˈrætɪk/ *adj.* likely to perform unpredictably 飘忽不定的；不稳定的
e.g. They no longer fear the erratic behavior of the market.

fissure /ˈfɪʃə/ *n.* a deep crack in something, especially in rock or in the ground 裂缝
e.g. Just ahead of us there was a huge fissure.

bandana /bænˈdænə/ *n.* a large and brightly colored handkerchief 印花大手帕
e.g. A bandana is good head protection and is an all-around useful item to have.

outside, this can be a big issue right now compared to those spending most, if not all, of their time indoors. Runners will likely be washing their hands more—which is good—but they may see more dryness and irritation as a result—especially with **erratic** spring weather thrown into the mix.

⑤ As the skin becomes dry, it can be irritated from inflammation, which can lead to itching, and then it will start to form small, painful nicks that can bleed and enlarge, and may lead to scratching, which will worsen skin cracking.

⑥ Micro-tears can evolve into deeper **fissures** this way, and then your protective barrier isn't so protective any more. You could be more susceptible to skin infections, as well as other germs, including viruses.

Skin Issues with Face Masks

⑦ First and foremost, a quick reminder is to reserve N95 masks for health care workers instead of DIY masks—including **bandanas** or scarves, as long as they can be washed immediately—when you go out in public. The purpose of the mask is not to protect you, but to protect other people from you. Even with cloth masks, though, skin can get irritated due to trapped moisture, and because you have to tie or loop the masks so they're firmly pressed against the face, that pressure can raise the likelihood of redness and sensitivity.

⑧ A good strategy after you've removed your mask using proper procedures (avoid touching the front of the mask, and wash your hands right afterward) is to wash your face. But be sure to wash your hands first so you're not transferring germs from the mask into your mouth, nose, and eyes.

9 Much like the hand **scrubbing**, more face washing can increase your chances of developing dry skin, especially in the areas around the nose and mouth, where the mask has been. Avoid the temptation to scratch or adjust your mask, or even reach under the mask and rub your nose subconsciously.

How to Boost Your Skin Health

10 There are ways to keep your hands and face from turning into a hot desert landscape. In general, creams contain more oil than water-based lotions, so they're more moisturizing and protective.

11 At night, you can start a routine that will lock in moisture as you sleep. The first step would be to use a gentle cleanser such as **micellar** water, and then to apply a thick cream-type moisturizer to your hands and face. If you just have moderate dryness, stop there.

12 Because coronavirus can remain on surfaces for at least a day—and on some types of surfaces for a few days, it's possible to pick them up on your hands and transfer them into your system by touching your mouth, nose, or eyes. The more barriers between you and coronavirus germs, the better.

New Words and Expressions

scrub /skrʌb/ *v.* to wash hard and thoroughly 用力擦洗
e.g. Although she scrubbed the old pot thoroughly, she could not make it look completely clean.

micellar /maɪˈselə/ *adj.* microcellular 胶束的；微胞的
e.g. This review deals with the recent progress on micellar catalysis.

(643 words)

(Source: Millard, E. 2020. How to Upgrade Your Skincare Routine During the Coronavirus Pandemic. 04–10. From Runner's World website.)

Read the text carefully and then complete the statements with appropriate words.

1. She's being _____ as the next leader of the party.

2. She passed her tongue over her _____ lips and tried to speak.

3. The new drug is a(n) _____ lifesaver.

4. He was a singer, but _____ a scholar.

5. The remaining 20 patients were _____ to another hospital.

6. Sexual contact is responsible for the bulk of HIV _____.

7. _____ behavior at home may be hard to handle.

8. All action begins with an intention, whether consciously or _____.

9. Once in the bloodstream, the bacteria _____ the surface of the red cells.

10. Overweight children are also _____ to developing the disorder.

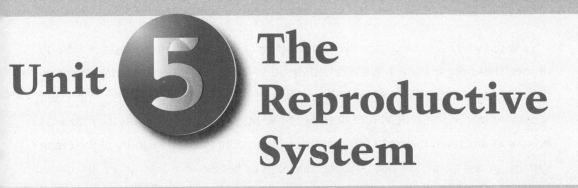

Unit 5

The Reproductive System

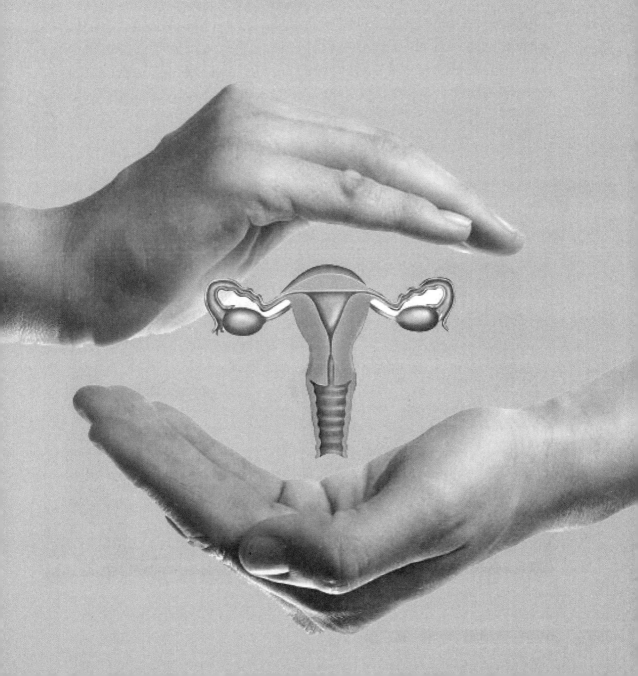

Pre-reading

As the very name suggests, the reproductive or genital system consists of a group of specialized organs which work in coordination for giving birth to human offspring through sexual means. Some non-living substances also come to play a very important accessory role in the proper functioning of the human reproductive system such as hormones and pheromones. It is quite surprising to note that the majority of the organ systems in one's body do not differ on the basis of gender, but here you will witness significant differences in males and females.

How does the magical fertilization happen? What is the mysterious circumcision and how is it performed? Is it possible to transplant the uterus from a deceased donor? How much do you know about HIV? What appropriate protective measures shall we take to prevent it? You may find out the answers in the following passages.

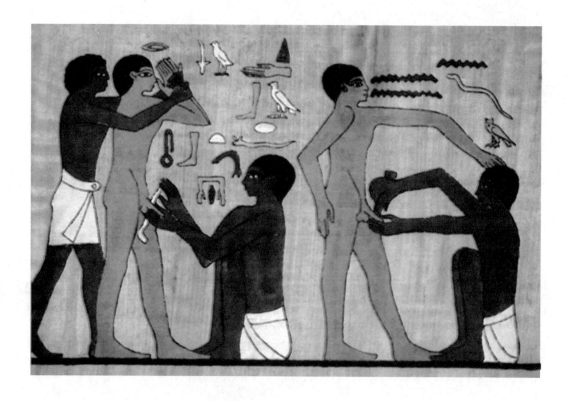

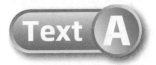

The Epic Journey—How Fertilization Happens

❶ While only a single egg is released each month, millions of sperms set off on a journey in a single ejaculation—all with their eye on that single prize. But only one of those sperms will be crowned the victor, and the chances are stacked against fertilization. Luckily, eggs and sperms have developed some pretty skillful tricks to give themselves a fighting chance.

Fortify the Troops

❷ The liquid portion of semen not only provides the sperms with nourishment for the journey, it also solidifies in a woman's vagina (阴道) after ejaculation, forming a physical barrier that prevents the sperms from wandering very far in the wrong direction. This protection disappears within half an hour, when the semen becomes a liquid. Any sperm that hasn't made it up through the cervix (子宫颈) by then is clearly not worth saving, and those left behind for more than a few moments don't have much of a chance anyway; the vagina is an acidic place to hang out

New Words and Expressions

ejaculation /ɪˌdʒækjʊˈleɪʃn/ *n.* the discharge of sperms in males 射精
e.g. Each male ejaculation will contain up to 300 million sperms.

semen /ˈsiːmən/ *n.* the liquid containing sperms that is produced by the sex organs of men and male animals 精液；精子
e.g. Interviews revealed that males with good semen quality ate more fruits and vegetables.

New Words and Expressions

thrash /θræʃ/ *v.* to move or stir about violently 猛烈摆动

　　e.g. She would thrash around in her hospital bed and remove her intravenous line.

ovary /ˈəʊvərɪ/ *n.* the two organs in a woman's body that produce eggs 卵巢

　　e.g. Ovarian cancer is a malignant tumor in the ovary.

and quickly destroys any errant cells (that's why sperms fall out of you after you have sex).

Call in the Transport Unit

❸　The cervical canal is a much more welcoming environment, and sperms that make it there find themselves awash in a sea of cervical mucus. This is also a good thing, since that mucus is specially designed to transport sperms efficiently when you're most fertile. As you approach ovulation (排卵期), your suddenly plentiful mucus becomes stretchy, clear, and thin (that's one of the reasons why observing it is such an effective method of determining your ovulation time). The changes happen at a microscopic level as well, as strings of molecules line up like train tracks so that sperms can hop on and ride to their destination.

Gather Steam

❹　Even sperms that are fearless enough to get this far aren't home free. A just-ejaculated sperm cell has to spend a couple of hours going through biochemical changes, picking up tail-**thrashing** speed as it makes its way into the uterus and fallopian (输卵管) tubes to find its target.

Check the Coordinates

❺　The biggest key to successful fertilization is timing. Sperms must reach their destination—the egg (which is slowly making its way down the fallopian tube from your **ovary**)—within the right time frame. If they get there too early, they risk dying before the egg shows up. Too late, the egg will be gone and they'll have missed their shot, so to speak. They also need to pick their destination carefully: An egg is usually only present in one of your two fallopian tubes in any given month. Pick the wrong tube, and the sperms end up hanging out partying together with no guest of honor in sight.

Battle to the Finish

⑥　Even the sperms who reach the egg still have their work cut out for them. The race is on to be the first one to plow through the hard outer layer of the egg. And there's plenty of competition. Hundreds of sperms will surround the egg during the frantic battle to the finish, all trying to penetrate the egg's membrane to reach the cytoplasm (细胞质), where the sperm will then release its own genetic contribution. May the best sperm win!

Mission Accomplished

⑦　As soon as one lucky sperm cell succeeds in penetrating the egg, the egg immediately undergoes a chemical reaction that prevents other sperm cells from penetrating as well. Then the **chromosomes** carried by the sperm and egg come together, and the egg is officially fertilized. Within a matter of hours, the microscopic zygote (受精卵) divides, then divides again and again. About a week later, a ball of around 100 cells [called a blastocyst (囊胚)] reaches your uterus and settles down into the uterine lining. You have now reached **implantation**—the moment that fertilization gives way to pregnancy—

New Words and Expressions

chromosome /ˈkrəʊməsəʊm/ *n.* a threadlike body in the cell nucleus that carries the genes in a linear order 染色体
e.g. The scientists want to locate the position of the gene on a chromosome.

implantation /ˌɪmplɑːnˈteɪʃn/ *n.* the attachment of the blastocyst of an embryo to the wall of the uterus of the mother （受精卵或胚胎）着床
e.g. While many consider fertilization to be the start of pregnancy, successful implantation is another crucial hurdle.

when the sperm's journey gives way to your own incredible, life-transforming trip to parenthood.

(642 words)

(Source: Reece, T. 2021. The Epic Journey—How Fertilization Happens. 04–06. From What to Expect website.)

Task One

Decide whether the following statements are true (T) or false (F) according to the text.

1. _____ Only a sperm is released each month.
2. _____ The liquid portion of semen prevents the sperms from wandering in the wrong direction.
3. _____ The cervical canal is an acidic place and quickly destroys any errant cells.
4. _____ Sperms must reach their destination—the egg as early as possible.
5. _____ When one sperm cell succeeds in penetrating the egg, others would lose the chance.

Task Two

Fill in the blanks with the words given below. Change their forms if necessary.

stack	fortify	semen	stretchy	errant
crown	frantic	membrane	awash	fertile

1. The odds are _____ against civilians getting a fair trial.
2. In rape cases the offender usually leaves _____.
3. Queen Elizabeth was _____ in 1952.
4. Water rushes in, and the _____ expands.
5. Now kids are _____ in orange and black clothes, face paint and hair dye.

6. It also helped _____ our market position online.

7. The operation cannot be reversed to make her _____ again. She will never have her own babies.

8. Tests showed these layers were _____, as strong as steel and almost transparent.

9. _____ advertising is a leading cause.

10. A bird had been locked in and was by now quite _____.

Task Three

Paraphrase the following sentences from Text A.

1. While only a single egg is released each month, millions of sperms set off on a journey in a single ejaculation—all with their eye on that single prize. (Para. 1)

_____

_____

_____

_____

2. The liquid portion of semen not only provides the sperms with nourishment for the journey, it also solidifies in a woman's vagina after ejaculation, forming a physical barrier that prevents the sperms from wandering very far in the wrong direction. (Para. 2)

_____

_____

_____

_____

3. Even sperms that are fearless enough to get this far aren't home free. (Para. 4)

_____

_____

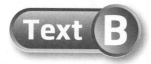

The Cutting Truth About Circumcision

New Words and Expressions

circumcision /ˌsɜːkəmˈsɪʒn/ *n.* the cutting off of the foreskin of males that is practiced as a religious rite by Jews and Muslims and by others as a social custom or for potential health benefits (such as improved hygiene) 割礼；净心；包皮环割术

e.g. There is no medical organization in the world that routinely recommends male infant circumcision.

❶ When was **circumcision** first practiced? How did it evolve? Why was it practiced? The earliest literary evidence of the practice of circumcision goes back to ancient Egypt.

❷ There are many hypotheses regarding the roots of the practice. Early Western scholars attributed the origins of circumcision to ancient Egypt. But many scholars today believe that the origin of the practice, as it is done in the West and the Middle East, goes back farther and originates with the inhabitants of southern Arabia and parts of Africa. Over the millennia, circumcision has been most often used as a religious rite, a rite of passage into manhood, but also as a form of punishment in wartime.

A Little or a Lot

❸ Circumcision has been practiced in parts of Africa, Oceania, and Jewish and Islamic countries. The form of circumcision that Westerners are most familiar with is complete removal of the foreskin or prepuce（包皮）, as it is practiced in Judaism. However, in ancient Egypt and other cultures in Africa, only part of the foreskin was removed. In the Pacific islands, the frenum（系带）was **snipped** but the foreskin was left untouched. This is interesting considering a Biblical reference where Jehovah commands the Israelites to circumcise their children again, "a second time". This could imply that some of them had already been circumcised in the Egyptian way and had to be circumcised in the Jewish or Israelite way.

Circumcision in Egypt and Israel

❹　In ancient Egypt, circumcision had a rather different function and process than it did in ancient Israel. In ancient Israel, circumcision was taken as a sign of membership in the **covenant** community established between God and Abraham. It was an ethnic marker showing that they were a part of the Israelite nation.

❺　Although it could be performed on adults if needed, it was usually performed on infants, eight days after birth, like among modern Jews. An adult was usually only circumcised if a non-Israelite decided that he wanted to be inducted into the Israelite community. Later, when the Israelite religion became more organized, becoming ancient Judaism, converts to Judaism were required to undergo circumcision. One way that early Christianity first distinguished itself from Judaism was that non-Jewish Christians were not required to be circumcised.

❻　In Egypt, it was typically done on adolescent

New Words and Expressions

snip /snɪp/ *v.* to sever or remove by pinching or clipping 剪断
e.g. He has now begun to snip away at the piece of paper.

covenant /ˈkʌvənənt/ *n.* a signed written agreement between two or more parties (nations) to perform some action 契约
e.g. We share an eternal covenant.

priesthood /ˈpriːsthʊd/ *n.* the position of being a priest or the period of time during which someone is a priest 教士（或神父、牧师、司铎）的职位；担任神职的时期

e.g. Should women be voted into the priesthood?

archaeological /ˌɑːkɪəˈlɒdʒɪkl/ *adj.* related to or dealing with or devoted to archaeology 考古学的

e.g. These archaeological findings are part of the national possessions.

elaborate /ɪˈlæbərɪt/ *adj.* containing a lot of careful details or many detailed parts（计划、系统、程序等）繁复的，详尽的，复杂的

e.g. They're making the most elaborate preparations for the wedding.

men who were about to be initiated into the **priesthood** or as adult males of the noble class. It is not clear that this is the case from **archaeological** and historical records, but Egyptian circumcision may also have been used to define a special elite class. Egyptian circumcision is depicted on temple walls where young men are seen being restrained as a priest performs the circumcision with a knife.

The Practice in Other African Cultures

❼ Egypt is not the only African culture that practiced or practices circumcision. It is common among East African peoples and the Bantu (班图人), usually as a rite of passage into manhood. Young males of the Xhosa (科萨人) and Zulu (祖鲁人) ethnic groups traditionally had an **elaborate** circumcision ritual where their bodies would be painted with whitewash before their circumcision.

❽ During the process, they would be isolated from the community for several weeks, especially from women. After the circumcision, they would abandon their cut foreskin in the forest, a symbol of them leaving behind their boyhood lives to become men, and then wash the whitewash off in a river. Circumcision is still regularly practiced among these cultures, but usually in hospitals instead of the traditional way.

Circumcision in Oceania

❾ Circumcision historically was not limited to only Africa and the Middle East. A form of circumcision was also practiced in Oceania and Aboriginal Australia using sea shells as the cutting instrument. Circumcision in Oceania and Australia was a rite of passage into manhood as well as a test of bravery.

❿ Circumcision is becoming increasingly controversial due to concerns about lack of informed consent and **infringement** of human rights.

New Words and Expressions

infringement /ɪnˈfrɪndʒmənt/ *n.* an act that disregards an agreement or a right 侵犯；违反
e.g. There might have been an infringement of the rules.

(647 words)

(Source: Strom, C. 2018. The Cutting Truth About Circumcision. 07–19. From Ancient Origins website.)

Task

Text B has ten paragraphs. Choose the correct summary for each of them from the list below.

List of Paragraph Summaries

1.	Adults got circumcised for social and religious reasons.
2.	Circumcision is the subject of intense public arguments.
3.	Answers to questions about circumcision go back to Ancient Egypt.
4.	Functions and processes of circumcision differed in Egypt and Israel.
5.	Circumcision was also performed in Oceania and Aboriginal Australia.
6.	Other African cultures besides Egypt also performed circumcision.
7.	There are hypotheses regarding the origin of circumcision.
8.	There are different forms of circumcision in different places.

9.	Men would be separated from others before circumcision and the cut foreskin would be thrown away.
10.	In Egypt, circumcision was practiced on teenager men who were going to be priests or men of the noble class.

Para. 1		Para. 2		Para. 3		Para. 4		Para. 5	
Para. 6		Para. 7		Para. 8		Para. 9		Para. 10	

Post-reading

The First Successful Uterus Transplant from a Deceased Donor

New Words and Expressions

feat /fiːt/ *n.* a notable achievement 功绩，壮举
e.g. A racing car is an extraordinary feat of engineering.

❶ A Brazilian baby will celebrate her first birthday today, less than two years after her mother—unable to carry a pregnancy because she lacked a uterus—underwent a transplant from a deceased donor. The mother is the first in the world to give birth after such a transplant, a **feat** doctors were not sure would ever be possible.

❷ The baby girl is healthy and developing normally, according to Dani Ejzenberg, the doctor at the University of Sao Paulo in Brazil who led the transplant team.

❸ For years researchers have been trying to help women who had been either born without uteruses or lost them for medical reasons to carry their own children. About a dozen babies have now been born from uteruses provided by living donors—usually the recipient's mother, sister, or friend—out of about 50 attempts worldwide. In 2011, a team in Turkey was the first to transplant a uterus from a deceased donor, but the procedure did not lead to a live birth.

❹ Ejzenberg says that attempt inspired him to begin a program in Brazil. He traveled to Sweden to learn from doctors there who have the most experience with uterine transplantation. He also tried the procedure on a second Brazilian woman, but she had to have the uterus removed two days after the operation because of complications. Two more women in his program are awaiting suitable donors.

❺ In the successful case, the donor was a 45-year-old mother of three who died from a rare type of stroke, and also donated her heart, liver, and kidneys. The unnamed uterus recipient was a 32-year-old woman born without a uterus, but otherwise healthy.

❻ The transplant was performed on September 20, 2016, and a fertilized embryo was implanted about seven months later. The baby was born by **cesarean** section between 34 and 36 weeks. Several of the Swedish women who had received uteruses from living donors experienced complications

> **New Words and Expressions**
>
> **cesarean** /sɪˈzeərɪən/ *n.* (also called C-section) the delivery of a fetus by surgical incision through the abdominal wall and uterus (from the belief that Julius Caesar was born that way) 剖腹产手术；剖宫产术
> **e.g.** Unless absolutely necessary, I would like to avoid a cesarean.

from the immunosuppressive medication needed to keep their bodies from rejecting the transplant.

❼ The Brazilian woman did not have any pregnancy problems, but the doctor removed the uterus during the C-section because he wanted to focus on helping more women have a single child rather than on one woman having more than one. For future procedures, he hopes to cut down on the time by removing the uterus before other organs, like the heart and kidneys. A research team has shown other organs do not suffer if the uterus is removed first.

❽ These are still early days for uterine transplants. It is not clear yet, for instance, whether transplants from live or deceased donors will end up being more successful in the long run.

❾ With a living donor, the surgery can be scheduled when it's convenient for the surgeons, and there is time to do a thorough assessment of the donated organ to make sure it is suitable. With a deceased donor, things are a little more rushed and the timing might not be ideal, but surgeons can take more tissue from the vagina and blood vessel network than is possible with a living donor.

❿ Another unknown is how likely the body is to reject a transplanted uterus, and thus how much anti-rejection medication the recipient would need. Each organ type triggers a different level of immune response, and because the uterus is only needed for a short time—rather than a lifetime, as with a kidney or heart—patients may be able to get away with less medication. The drugs have triggered pregnancy complications in some of the Swedish patients, including kidney problems and pre-eclampsia (先兆子痫).

⓫ Three teams in the US are now working on uterine transplants. Baylor has had two successful births from live donations; Cleveland Clinic is working toward deceased donations; and her own program will be performing both living and deceased donor transplants over the next year. Uterine transplantation began in other countries where there are legal or ethical barriers to **surrogacy**—getting someone else to carry the pregnancy.

⓬ The work on transplantation is important both as an option for **infertile** couples and to increase scientific understanding of the uterus and pregnancy.

> ### New Words and Expressions
>
> **surrogacy** /ˈsʌrəgəsɪ/ *n.* an arrangement by which a woman gives birth to a baby on behalf of another woman who is physically unable to have babies herself, and then gives the baby to her 代孕
> **e.g.** In this country, it is illegal to pay for surrogacy.
>
> **infertile** /ɪnˈfɜːtaɪl/ *adj.* incapable of reproducing 不能生殖的；不毛的；不结果实的；不肥沃的
> **e.g.** New medical techniques provide hope for infertile patients.

(683 words)

(Source: Weintraub, K. 2018. First Successful Uterus Transplant from a Deceased Donor. 12–05. From Scientific American website.)

Your reading time: _____ mins

Your reading rate: _____ words/min

Read the text as quickly as you can and then choose the best answer to each question.

1. Which of the following statements is true about the Brazilian baby's mother?

    A. She's the first woman to have a transplanted uterus.

    B. She's the first woman who gave birth to a deceased baby.

    C. She's the first woman with a transplanted uterus from the deceased donor and gave birth to a baby.

    D. She's the first woman to be a uterus donor.

2. Which of the following is not the group whom researchers have been trying to help?

    A. Women who have been born without uteruses.

    B. Women who have lost uteruses for medical reasons.

    C. Women who have done illegal abortion.

    D. Women who have always expected to carry a baby.

3. Which of the following statements is true according to the text?

    A. More than ten babies have been born from uteruses provided by living donors.

    B. Donors must be the recipient's relatives.

    C. The transplants from living donors are more successful in the long run.

    D. Patients of uterus transplantation may get away with little medication.

4. What does Para. 9 tell us?

    A. Transplantation from living donors is easier.

    B. Transplantation from living donors gives doctors more time for thorough assessment.

    C. Transplantation from deceased donors is easier.

    D. Transplantation from deceased donors gives doctors more time for the operation.

5. Which of the following facts is not the reason why transplantation from deceased donors is hard?

    A. Doctors cannot choose the most suitable time.

    B. Doctors cannot do thorough examinations.

C. It's unknown how likely the body is to reject a transplanted uterus.

D. Surgeons can take more tissue from the vagina and blood vessel network than is possible with a living donor.

Your comprehension rate: _____ %

Additional Reading

Everyone Should Know About HIV

1 Here are eight things you should know about HIV that can help you remain healthy and happy for many years to come, whether you are infected or not.

Early Detection and Early Treatment

2 Understanding the signs and symptoms of HIV allows us to proactively treat (and even avoid) certain infections well before they occur. It's important to note, however, that there are often no symptoms at the onset of HIV infection, and that when symptoms finally do appear, it's often after the virus has caused irreparable damage to a person's immune system.

3 Fear and misconceptions about HIV can often prevent people from seeking the treatment and care they need, with some misinterpreting the term "asymptomatic" as meaning "without

New Words and Expressions

abatement /əˈbeɪtmənt/ *n.* an interruption in the intensity or amount of something 减少；消除；减轻
e.g. The problem has persisted for about three or four weeks now, with no sign of abatement.

avert /əˈvɜːt/ *v.* to prevent the occurrence of something 避免，防止；转移
e.g. He did his best to avert suspicion.

infectivity /ɪnˈfektɪvɪtɪ/ *n.* the ability of a pathogen to establish an infection 传染性（影响别人）；易传染
e.g. The infectivity and other properties of viruses can be tested by several methods.

infection". Others, meanwhile, ignore the early symptoms until they eventually subside, failing to realize that the **abatement** of short-term symptoms is neither an indication of improvement nor the "all clear" sign that an infection has been **averted**.

Treatment on a Diagnosis Increases Life Expectancy

❹ On September 30, 2015, the World Health Organization revised its global HIV treatment guidelines to recommend the immediate initiation of antiretroviral (抗逆转录病毒的) therapy (ART) at the time of the diagnosis. According to the landmark Strategic Timing of Antiretroviral Treatment (START) study, treatment on a diagnosis not only increases the likelihood of a normal life span, but it also reduces the risk of HIV- and non-HIV-related illness by more than 50%. This is true irrespective of your age, sexual orientation, location, income, or immune status.

HIV Testing Is for Everyone

❺ The US Preventive Services Task Force (USPSTF) issued recommendations that all persons between the ages of 15 and 65 be screened for HIV as part of a routine doctor visit. The recommendations were made in line with evidence showing that early initiation of antiretroviral therapy will result in fewer HIV- and non-HIV-associated illnesses, as well as reduce the **infectivity** of a person with HIV.

In-home HIV Tests Work

6 In July 2012, the US Food and Drug Administration (FDA) granted approval to the OraQuick In-Home HIV Test, providing consumers with the first, over-the-counter oral HIV test able to provide confidential results in as little as 20 minutes. The FDA approval was welcomed by many community-based organizations, which have long cited the benefits of in-home testing at a time when 20% of the 1.2 million Americans infected with HIV are fully unaware of their status.

HIV Therapy Can Reduce Your Risk to Zero

7 Treatment as prevention (or TasP) is an evidence-based approach by which HIV-infected persons with an undetectable viral load are far less likely to transmit the virus to an uninfected (or untreated) partner. Current research has shown that achieving and maintaining an undetectable viral load altogether eliminates the risk of transmitting HIV to an uninfected partner.

PrEP Can Help You Avoid HIV

8 Pre-exposure prophylaxis (PrEP) is an HIV prevention strategy whereby the daily use of antiretroviral medication is known to significantly reduce a person's risk of acquiring HIV by anywhere from 75% to 92%. The evidence-based approach is considered an important part of an overall HIV prevention strategy, which includes the continued consistent use

New Words and Expressions

prophylaxis /ˌprɒfɪˈlæksɪs/ *n.* action that is taken in order to prevent disease 预防

e.g. This is known as drug prophylaxis.

New Words and Expressions

condom /ˈkɒndəm/ *n.* a thin rubber bag that a man wears over his penis during sex to prevent a woman having a baby or to protect against disease 避孕套
e.g. Most condoms are highly effective in preventing HIV and certain other sexually transmitted diseases.

conceive /kənˈsiːv/ *v.* to become pregnant 怀孕
e.g. She is unable to conceive.

irrefutable /ˌɪrɪˈfjuːtəbl/ *adj.* impossible to deny or disprove 无可辩驳的
e.g. The pictures provide irrefutable evidence of the incident.

of **condoms** and a reduction in the number of sexual partners. PrEP is not intended to be used in isolation.

Safe Pregnancy Is Possible

❾ According to the United Nations Joint Programme on HIV/AIDS (UNAIDS), nearly half of all HIV-affected couples in the world are serodiscordant, meaning that one partner is HIV-positive while the other is HIV-negative.

❿ In the United States alone, there are over 140,000 serodiscordant heterosexual couples, a great many of whom are of child-bearing age.

⓫ With major advances in antiretroviral therapy, as well as other preventative interventions, couples, of which one partner is living with HIV and the other is not, have far greater opportunities to **conceive** than ever before—allowing for pregnancy while minimizing the risk of transmission to both the child and uninfected partner.

Condoms Are as Important as Ever

⓬ Despite this being an age when HIV drugs are known to reduce the risk of transmission, both for uninfected people and those living with the disease, one fact remains **irrefutable**: Condoms remain the single most effective means of preventing HIV today.

(689 words)

(Source: Myhre, J. & Sifris, D. 2021. The 9 Things Everyone Should Know About HIV. 02–08. From Verywell Health website.)

Task

Read the text carefully and then complete the statements with appropriate words.

1. Having knowledge of HIV allows us to _____ treat certain infections.
2. Fear and _____ stop people from taking appropriate measures.
3. Life _____ can be increased if patients are treated well.
4. Treatment on a diagnosis _____ the risk of illness.
5. With advances in medical technology, serodiscordant couples have far greater opportunities to _____.
6. Using a condom is the _____ most effective means of preventing HIV.
7. People feel little sensation or change in their body at the _____ of HIV infection.
8. With FDA approval, consumers can have a(n) _____ oral HIV test at home.
9. The risk of _____ HIV can be reduced by daily use of antiretroviral medication.
10. The _____ approach is considered an important part of the strategy.

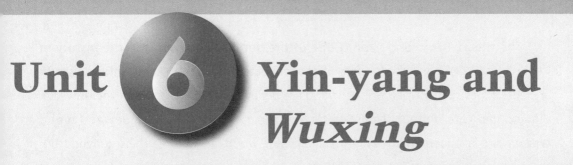

Unit 6 Yin-yang and *Wuxing*

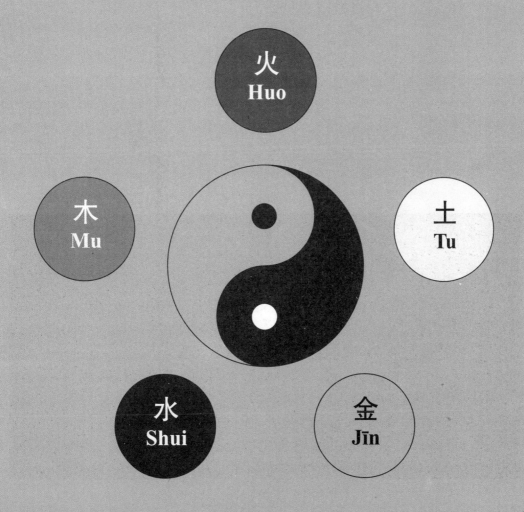

Pre-reading

The theory of yin and yang is one of the dominant concepts in the history of Chinese philosophy and the fundamental concept to both Taoism and Confucianism. In ancient Chinese philosophy, yin and yang are believed to be the origin of the universe. Yin and yang are mutual opposites such as the sun and the moon, day and night. *Wuxing* (the Five Elements), namely metal, water, wood, fire, and earth, is derived from these two components. The Five Elements are also the major foundation of traditional Chinese medicine. Whenever the elements experience imbalance, diseases will arise.

How are yin and yang applied in traditional Chinese medicine? How are yin and yang related to hormonal balance? What are the yin-yang and *Wuxing* qualities of different organs? You may find out the answers in the following passages.

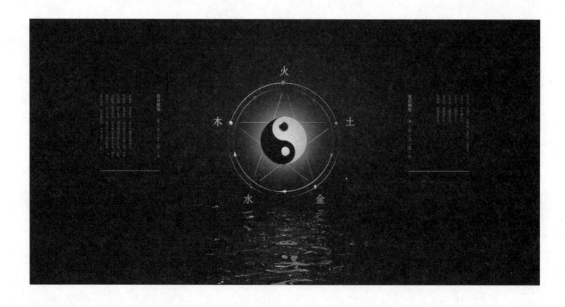

In-reading

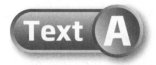

Yin-yang and *Wuxing* in Chinese Culture

❶   In ancient Chinese **cosmology**, the whole universe was believed to be **undifferentiated** and presented oneness. This is Tai Chi, the beginning of the cosmos. Gradually, yin and yang evolved out of Tai Chi. Yang is about releasing energy, which represents those that are upward, active, bright, expanding, **extroverted**, masculine, and lively. Yin is about contracting energy, which is downward, passive, dark, accumulated, **introverted**, feminine, and quiet. Everything in the world has both yin and yang sides and they are in constant motion and mutual transformation. The motion of yin and yang, then, generates the Four Images. The transitions between yin and yang are the lesser yin and lesser yang. All lives are born out of and come back to the earth; four seasons change under the moon and the sun. So, the moon and the sun together constitute Tai Chi, which contains both yin and yang; it corresponds to the earth on the ground. Then, *Wuxing* is formed.

New Words and Expressions

cosmology /kɒzˈmɒlədʒɪ/ *n.* a theory about the origin and nature of the Universe 宇宙论
e.g. Matter plays a central role in cosmology.

undifferentiated /ˌʌndɪfəˈrenʃɪeɪtɪd/ *adj.* having no distinguishing features 无差别的
e.g. By now, everyone is increasingly interconnected and undifferentiated.

extroverted /ˈekstrəvɜːtɪd/ *adj.* very active, lively, and friendly 外向的
e.g. He's extremely extroverted.

introverted /ˈɪntrəvɜːtɪd/ *adj.* shy, quiet, and preferring to spend time alone rather than often being with other people 内向的，不爱交际的
e.g. When she started school, she became cautious and introverted.

New Words and Expressions

erosion /ɪˈrəʊʒn/ *n.* the gradual destruction and removal of rock or soil in a particular area by rivers, the sea, or the weather 侵蚀
e.g. Soil erosion was mitigated by the planting of trees.

dike /daɪk/ *n.* a thick wall that is built to stop water flooding onto very low-lying land from a river or from the ocean 堤坝
e.g. When the river dike is completed, the crops will be safe against floods.

pictogram /ˈpɪktəɡræm/ *n.* a picture representing a word or phrase 象形图
e.g. The Chinese pictogram for "rain" depicted a raining scene.

diagram /ˈdaɪəɡræm/ *n.* a simple drawing which consists mainly of lines and is used, for example, to explain how a machine works 示意图
e.g. Like any such diagram, it is a simplification.

❷　The *Wuxing* Theory (the Five Elements Theory) is a philosophical term in ancient Chinese culture, which defines the nature and attributes of everything in the universe and its movements. The wood, fire, metal, water, and earth are five specific representatives or symbols of the Five Elements. The only permanent thing is changing. Therefore, all the elements in the universe are in constant motion, which constitutes interactions between the Five Elements. They can create or overcome one another. On the one hand, branches can create fire; burnt ashes become earth; metal ores are formed inside the earth; melted metal will be liquid and water nourishes wooden plants; on the other hand, metal tools can cut off plants; roots of trees grow inside of the earth and prevent soil **erosion**; **dikes** and dams can stop the flood; water can put out a fire and fire melts metal into liquid.

❸　It's quite possible that the ancient Chinese cosmology was more of collective intelligence; however, there are some famous kings that are related to the invention of this theory. Fu Xi (伏羲), an honorable king from around 5,000 years ago, used to observe the universe, trying to figure out a general rule. Soon, he got two **pictograms** [named He Tu Luo Shu (河图洛书)] from mythical creatures, from which he concluded yin and yang, Five Elements, and Eight **Diagrams** (*Bagua*). In *The Book of Documents* and *The Book of Changes*, the theory was mentioned. These two ancient books were written and preserved in some ancient royal places, and then organized and edited by Confucius centuries later.

❹ In traditional Chinese medicine and food therapy, a human's body is considered a complete cycle, which contains a whole system of yin and yang and the Five Elements. Important organs, emotions, and food all correspond to the Five Elements, based on their different attributes. Emotion and diet may influence certain organs with the same attributes. Therefore, the balance of yin and yang and the **neutralization** of the Five Elements are the essence of Chinese medicine and food therapy. Take "wood" for instance: in spring, or when someone's eye, liver, or gallbladder feels uncomfortable, or for irritable people, it's good to eat sour flavored or green colored food.

❺ Nowadays, many Chinese parents still name their babies based on the Five Elements Theory. Since the Heavenly Stems and Earthly Branches (天干地支) is the counting system of the Chinese calendar, based on a person's birth year, month, date, and hour, one's Five Elements' attribute can be calculated. In order to balance the Five Elements, parents would use Chinese characters that have the baby's least attribute. For instance, if someone has no or few elements of fire, he or she can use Chinese characters with the fire part in his or her name.

New Words and Expressions

neutralization /ˌnjuːtrəlaɪˈzeɪʃn/ *n.*
the action of making something chemically neutral 中和
e.g. Slowing digestion may allow more complete mixing of food and neutralization of acid.

(615 words)

(Source: Anon. 2019. Yin-yang and *Wuxing* in Chinese Culture. 04–11. From China Fetching website.)

Task One

Decide whether the following statements are true (T) or false (F) according to the text.

1. _____ Tai Chi is believed to be the beginning of the cosmos.

2. _____ In the universe, certain things have the yin side, while the others have the yang side.

3. _____ The theory of yin and yang defines the attributes of everything in the universe and its movements.

4. _____ The Five Elements only interact with each other through creation.

5. _____ If a child lacks the element water, he or she can be named with Chinese characters containing the water part to achieve balance and neutralization.

Task Two

Fill in the blanks with the words given below. Change their forms if necessary.

release	extroverted	constant	transition	constitute
correspond	erosion	collective	irritable	calculate

1. Testing patients without their consent would _____ a professional and legal offence.

2. The action of _____ can create different kinds of coastal landscape features.

3. Some young people who were easy-going and _____ as children become self-conscious in early adolescence.

4. Your account of events does not _____ with hers.

5. Inflation is a(n) _____ threat to the economy.

6. He had been waiting for over an hour and was beginning to feel _____.

7. He was _____ from custody the next day.

8. This formula is used to _____ the area of a circle.

9. This is a(n) _____ decision made by the whole village.

10. The _____ from school to work can be difficult.

Task Three

Paraphrase the following sentences from Text A.

1. Everything in the world has both yin and yang sides and they are in constant motion and mutual transformation. (Para. 1)

_____

_____

_____

_____

2. The only permanent thing is changing. (Para. 2)

_____

_____

_____

3. Important organs, emotions, and food all correspond to the Five Elements, based on their different attributes. (Para. 4)

_____

_____

_____

_____

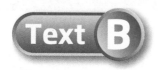

The Philosophy and Theory of Yin and Yang

New Words and Expressions

interdependence /ˌɪntədɪˈpendəns/

n. the condition of a group of people or things that all depend on each other 互相依赖

e.g. By accepting our interdependence and seeking to learn from each other, we will all benefit.

❶ The earliest reference to yin and yang is in *The Book of Changes* in approximately 700 BC. In this work, all phenomena are said to be reduced to yin and yang. The theory of yin and yang is one of the most fundamental concepts in traditional Chinese medicine, as it is the foundation of a diagnosis and treatment.

❷ There are four main aspects of yin and yang relationship:

- Yin and yang are opposites. They are either on the opposite ends of a cycle, like the seasons of a year, or, opposites on a continuum of energy or matter. This opposition is relative, and can only be spoken of in relationships. For example, water is yin relative to steam but yang relative to ice. Yin and yang are never static but in a constantly changing balance.

- Yin and yang cannot exist without each other. The Tai Chi diagram shows the relationship of yin and yang and illustrates **interdependence** of yin and yang. Nothing is totally yin or totally yang. Just as a state of total yin is reached, yang begins to grow. Yin contains the seed of yang and vice versa. They constantly transform into each other.

- Mutual consumption of yin and yang. Relative levels of yin and yang are continuously changing. Normally, this is a **harmonious** change, but when yin or yang is out of balance, they affect each other, and too much of one can eventually weaken (consume) the other.

- Inter-transformation of yin and yang. One can change into the other, but it is not a random event, happening only when the time is right. For example, spring only comes when winter is finished.

New Words and Expressions

vice versa /ˌvaɪs ˈvɜːsə/ used to say that the opposite of a situation you have just described is also true 反之亦然
e.g. Teachers qualified to teach in England are not accepted in Scotland, and vice versa.

harmonious /hɑːˈməʊnɪəs/ *adj.* arranged together in a pleasing way so that each part goes well with the others 和谐的，协调的
e.g. The architecture is harmonious and no building is over five or six floors high.

❸ The yin-yang theory is the fundamental principle and the most important theory in traditional Chinese medicine underlying all physiology, pathology, and treatment. Yin and yang had been understood for many centuries but were systematically elaborated and written down by Zou Yan of the Yin-yang (Naturalist) School in the Warring States Period (475–221 BC). The *Wuxing* Theory was developed at the same time. The Naturalist School promoted the idea of living in harmony with natural laws. Scholars of this school interpreted natural phenomena and observed how these are reflected in the human body in health and disease. Yin and yang and the Five Elements became an integral part of Chinese philosophy.

❹ All physiological processes, signs, and symptoms can be reduced to yin and yang. In general, every treatment modality aims to: **tonify** yang; tonify yin; **disperse** excess yang; disperse excess yin. Clinical signs and symptoms can be interpreted via the yin-yang theory. When yin and yang are in dynamic balance and relating harmoniously, there are no symptoms to observe. When yin and yang are out of balance, they become separated. For example, yin does not cool and nourishes yang so yang rises (headaches, red face, sore eyes, sore throats, nosebleeds, irritability, **manic** behavior); yang does not warm and activates yin (cold limbs, hypo-activity, poor circulation of blood, pale face, low energy). In medicine also, yin and yang transform into one another, but only when conditions are right. The right moment is determined by the internal qualities of the given situation or phenomenon. In clinical practice, the above principle is important.

❺ Diseases are prevented by achievement of balance in the lifestyle. For instance, excessive work (yang) without rest leads to deficiency (yin) of energy, excessive consumption of cold food (yin) leads to deficiency of the body's yang energy, and smoking (putting heat or yang into lungs) leads to deficiency of yin of lungs (and eventually kidneys). The principle is observable in pathological changes found in diseases. Exterior cold (cold weather) can invade the body and can change to heat (a sore throat), which is deficiency of yang of spleen. Because spleen yang is used to transform fluids, these can build up to cause excess interior dampness (yin).

(641 words)

(Source: Carina. 2018. The Philosophy and Theory of Yin and Yang. 03–20. From Cara Health website.)

Task

Text B has five paragraphs. Choose the correct summary for each of them from the list below.

List of Paragraph Summaries

1.	All clinical symptoms can be explained and treated according to the theory of yin and yang.
2.	The theory of yin and yang constitutes an essential concept in traditional Chinese medicine.
3.	The yin-yang relationship can be understood in four aspects.
4.	To maintain the balance of yin and yang is vital to the prevention of diseases.
5.	The theories of yin and yang and the Five Elements advocate living in harmony.

Para. 1		Para. 2		Para. 3		Para. 4		Para. 5	

Post-reading

The Yin and Yang of Hormonal Balance

New Words and Expressions

insomnia /ɪnˈsɒmnɪə/ *n.* habitual sleeplessness or inability to sleep 失眠

e.g. Depression is almost always accompanied by insomnia.

libido /lɪˈbiːdəʊ/ *n.* the part of the personality that is considered to cause the emotional, especially sexual desires 性欲

e.g. Lack of sleep is a major factor in loss of libido.

progesterone /prəʊˈdʒestərəʊn/ *n.* a hormone that is produced in the ovaries of women and female animals and helps prepare the body for pregnancy 孕酮；黄体酮

e.g. The drugs block the action of progesterone.

❶ Hormones are chemical messengers that influence the way our cells and organs function. There are many different types of hormones in the body and although each has a different function, they are all influenced by another. Hormones are produced, stored, and secreted via a network of glands, which make up our endocrine system. They control growth, development, reproduction, metabolism, mood, sleep, and digestion. When the body produces too much or little of a certain hormone, it is known as hormonal imbalance. Depending on the hormone(s) involved, a woman will experience a range of symptoms including moodiness, weight gain, digestive problems, acne, menstrual irregularities, infertility, headaches, **insomnia**, breast pain, anxiety, food cravings, and loss of **libido**.

❷ In traditional Chinese medicine, hormonal balance is closely tied to the concept of yin and yang balance. Although yin and yang are opposite in nature, they depend on one another to function properly. Hormonal balance occurs when yin and yang interchange smoothly, making room for change and transformation. Just as it is important for estrogen and **progesterone** to be balanced, so should the yin-yang ratio be balanced. If there is too much or too little yin or yang in the body, imbalance will occur, which leads to hormonal imbalance.

❸ Hormonal imbalance does not happen overnight. It takes time before symptoms become apparent. A **sedentary** person who sits too much and has a poor diet is likely to end up with heaviness and congestion (too much yin) in the lower part of his or her body. When blood cannot circulate properly and there is a buildup of fluids (not enough yang to move yin), problems such as sore back, varicose veins, achy legs, piles, and painful periods may occur. When the liver which is intimately connected to hormone balance, becomes congested, it will not be able to function properly. If the liver cannot process or biotransform hormones efficiently, the body will feel "out of balance", leading to hormonal imbalance. A woman who exercises too much without sufficient rest (too much yang) will end up putting so much stress on her body; she will drain her reserves. When a person's reserves which are stored in kidneys and **adrenals**, are running low, symptoms such as tiredness, low libido, and poor appetite are common. If the body produces a lower than normal level of hormones (yin deficiency), it can lead to hormonal imbalance. This, in turn, may lead to **amenorrhea** (no periods) or infertility due to ovulation problems.

❹ The goal of traditional Chinese medicine is to restore balance in the body. Acupuncture and herbal medicine are safe and effective forms

New Words and Expressions

sedentary /ˈsedəntrɪ/ *adj.* (of a person) tending to spend much time being seated 久坐的
e.g. Obesity and a sedentary lifestyle have been linked with an increased risk of heart disease.

adrenal /əˈdriːnl/ *n.* either of a pair of complex endocrine glands situated near the kidney 肾上腺
e.g. Tumors had spread to his back, spine, and adrenal gland.

amenorrhea /eɪˌmenəˈriːə/ *n.* absence or suppression of normal menstruation 闭经；月经不调
e.g. The reason for primary amenorrhea is very complicated.

New Words and Expressions

cruciferous /kruːˈsɪfərəs/ *adj.* relating to or denoting plants of the cabbage family 十字花科的

e.g. Broccoli, cauliflower, and cabbage are all part of the cruciferous vegetable family.

of treatments, which promote a healthy balance. Acupuncture has a regulating effect on the body and herbs have a hormone balancing effect on the body. They both play an important role in regulating the menstrual cycle, balancing emotions and promoting healthy organ function.

5 During a consultation, a traditional Chinese medicine practitioner will inquire about your general state of health and examine your tongue and pulse. Depending on your yin-yang ratio and accompanying symptoms, he or she will select the most appropriate treatment for you. He or she will also advise you on the best diet, form of exercise, and supplements to support you.

6 Some general recommendations are as follows:

- Eat organic foods and hormone-free meats where possible.

- Add more cabbage, broccoli, Brussel sprouts, and cauliflower to your diet. These **cruciferous** vegetables help break down estradiol (a form of estrogen) in the body. Too much estradiol can contribute to breast pain, weight gain, moodiness, low libido, breast and uterine cancer.

- Eliminate caffeine, nicotine, and alcohol.

- Avoid junk food.

- Take time out to do things you like—hikes, facials, pedicures, foot massage, book reading, and meditation.

- Zinc, magnesium (镁), vitamin B_6, and vitamin C are helpful.

(624 words)

(Source: Buonocore, G. 2019. The Yin and Yang of Hormonal Balance. 01–24. From IMI website.)

Your reading time: _____ mins

Your reading rate: _____ words/min

Task

Read the text as quickly as you can and then choose the best answer to each question.

1. What can be inferred about hormones according to the text?

    A. Different hormones may have similar functions.

    B. Different hormones function independently.

    C. Hormones are produced through a network of glands.

    D. Hormones cannot exert an influence on the digestion process.

2. Which of the following will not lead to hormonal imbalance?

    A. Too much of a certain hormone.

    B. Too little of a certain hormone.

    C. An imbalanced yin-yang ratio.

    D. A balanced estrogen and progesterone level.

3. What might happen to a woman who sits too much and has a poor diet?

    A. She may end up with too much yin building up in the upper part of her body.

    B. Her blood circulation will not be affected.

C. She may suffer from achy legs.

D. Her stomach will become congested.

4. Which of the following statements is false about traditional Chinese medicine treatment for hormonal imbalance?

A. The patient's temperature will be taken during consultation.

B. The goal is to restore balance in the body.

C. Acupuncture and herbal medicine can help restore balance in the body.

D. An appropriate treatment will be selected based on the patient's yin-yang ratio and symptoms.

5. What should a person do to maintain hormonal balance?

A. To exercise more.

B. To quit smoking.

C. To eat foods with hormones.

D. To eat vegetables with estradiol.

Your comprehension rate: _____ %

Additional Reading

Understanding Organs with the Yin-yang and *Wuxing* Theory

New Words and Expressions

axiomatic /ˌæksɪəˈmætɪk/ *adj.*
(formal) true in such an obvious way that you do not need to prove it 不言而喻的；不证自明的
e.g. It is axiomatic that life is not always easy.

❶ It is **axiomatic** that within yang there is yin, and within yin there is yang. The five organs have different yin-yang qualities. The lung is a yin-predominant metal organ. The yin of lung metal gathers fluids and *qi*, which fills the body; the yang of lung metal divides fluids and *qi* into clear and **turbid**. Lung metal thus gathers dampness, separates fluids into clear and turbid, and thereby creates kidney water.

❷　The kidney is a yin-predominant water organ. The yin of kidney water holds water and lubricates the body. The yang of kidney water moves fluids and provides the body with strength. Kidney water yang supports the erectness of liver wood, and kidney water yin supports the flexibility of liver wood. Thus, kidney water yin and yang together create liver wood.

❸　The liver is a yang-predominant wood organ. The yang of liver wood provides the body with uprightness, so it can stand erect; the yin of liver wood provides flexibility, so the body can bend. The erectness of liver wood yang supports the floating/active yang of heart fire, while the flexibility of liver wood yin supports the calming/grounding yin of heart fire. Therefore, liver wood yin and yang together create heart fire.

❹　The heart is a yang-predominant fire organ. Remember that the spirit is yang and the body is yin. The heart is the abode of the spirit, and the spirit keeps a person alive. The yang of heart fire impels the spirit outward to make the person active during the day. The yin of heart fire holds or encloses the spirit and allows the body to rest during the night. The more a person becomes physically or mentally active, the more the body demands yin-yang *qi*, which allows

New Words and Expressions

turbid /ˈtɜːbɪd/ *adj.* full of mud, dirt, etc. so that you cannot see through it 混浊的；混乱的

e.g. How can we make this glass of turbid water clear?

consolidate /kən'sɒlɪdeɪt/ *v.* to make a position of power or success stronger so that it is more likely to continue 使加强
e.g. Italy consolidated their lead with a second goal.

edema /ɪ'diːmə/ *n.* an excessive accumulation of serous fluid in the intercellular spaces of tissue 浮肿
e.g. Is it true that heart failure can cause systemic edema?

spleen soil to transform food for the needs of the *Wuxing* organs. When the body is at rest, the requirement of yin-yang *qi* is less, which allows spleen soil to store. So the yin and yang of heart fire together create spleen soil.

❺ The spleen is a yin-predominant soil organ. The yin of spleen soil receives and stores food. The yang of spleen soil transforms food to provide for the yin-yang needs of the *Wuxing* organs. The receiving and storing yin nature of spleen soil allows lung metal to gather and **consolidate** *qi* and fluids; the sorting and transforming nature of the spleen soil allows lung metal to separate fresh and waste *qi* and fluids. Thus, the yin and yang of spleen soil together create lung metal.

❻ While lung metal creates kidney water, it also controls liver wood. Metal in the soil stabilizes wood, so that wood does not fall. Lung metal fills the body with *qi* that binds liver wood in place, so a person does not fall. While kidney water creates liver wood, it also controls heart fire, so a person is grounded while active. While liver wood creates heart fire, it also controls spleen soil. Wood holds soil, so there is no slipping of land. Spleen soil receives and distributes food. Liver wood holds spleen soil, so a person can stop intake of food when the *Wuxing* organs have sufficient yin-yang *qi*. While heart fire creates spleen soil, it also controls lung metal, so a person can breathe smoothly. While spleen soil creates lung metal, it also controls kidney water, so a person is moist but not flooded (e.g. **edema**).

❼ All human physical functions are maintained by the *Wuxing* organs. Lung metal governs the *qi* of the entire body. The yin of lung metal gathers moisture and *qi* from heaven, earth, and the *Wuxing* organs to fill the body. Like metal that divides water and **sludge**, the yang of lung metal separates to produce fresh *qi* and water, exhales waste *qi* through the mouth and nose, excretes body waste via the large intestine, and thus maintains the freshness and lightness of the body. Thus, all symptoms such as shortness of breath and fever indicate lung metal yin damage.

New Words and Expressions

sludge /slʌdʒ/ *n.* thick mud, sewage, or industrial waste 烂泥

e.g. At least, until the snow hardened into ice, the whiteness turned to sludge, and everyone started to moan again.

(660 words)

[Source: Chang, R. 2018. Understanding Organs with the Yin-yang and *Wuxing* Theory. *The Journal of Chinese Medicine*, (118): 10-11.]

Task

Read the text carefully and then complete the statements with appropriate words.

1. It is _____ that as people grow older, they generally become less agile.
2. The _____ symbol is a circle made up of black and white swirls, each containing a spot of the other.
3. Regular exercise strengthens the heart, _____ reducing the risk of heart attack.
4. He _____ the most ordinary subject into the sublime.
5. He tried to _____ his power by putting forth policies that moderately helped the lower classes.
6. Although her illness is serious, her condition is beginning to _____.
7. The company _____ the products within the country.

8. These reasons are not _____ to justify the ban.

9. _____ is a condition characterized by an excess of watery fluid collecting in the cavities or tissues of the body.

10. The skin _____ sweat.

Unit 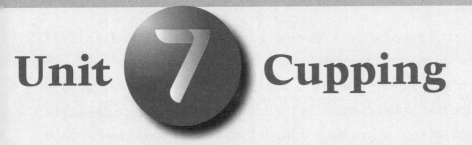 Cupping

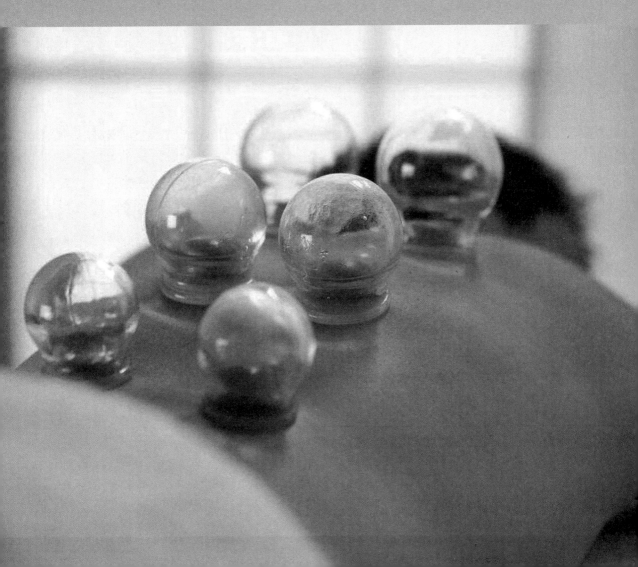

Pre-reading

The red scars on the back of the American swimmer Michael Phelps have drawn worldwide attention to a mysterious medicine in the East. That's cupping! Originated in ancient China, cupping is treasured as a therapeutic treatment to draw blood to the surface of the body through a glass vessel. It is based on the Chinese philosophy of health balance between *qi* (energy) and blood. With its amazingly detoxifying and relieving effect, cupping is widely used both in China and abroad.

How is it working? Is it more competitive than acupuncture? Is it horrible to see blood flowing onto the surface? The first three passages in this unit will present you the basic idea of the Oriental therapy with its merits and demerits, and the last passage may provide some food for thought from an academic perspective.

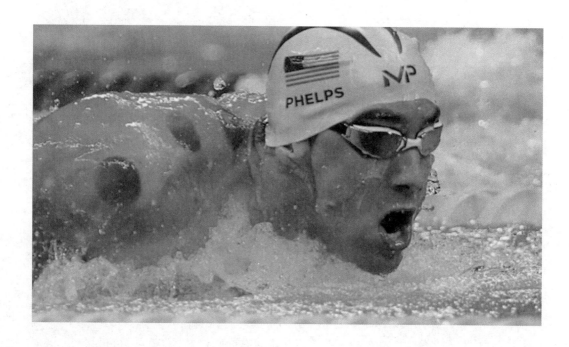

In-reading

Text A

The Secrets Behind Cupping Therapy

❶ Some old medical textbooks in the Western world described cupping therapy as a medical practice used by Egyptians to cure some frequent diseases. There have also been accounts of Hippocrates using the cupping method for internal diseases. Fire cupping has also been practiced throughout Europe, Asia, and Africa. Cupping therapy is an **alternative** form of medicine and is perhaps better known as a traditional Chinese medicine, like acupuncture.

❷ Cupping used to be performed using hollowed-out animal horns and was a method employed to treat boils, snakebites, and skin lesions. The cupping method was said to pull toxins from the body. The application of cupping, throughout the years, has evolved from the use of animal horns to bamboo cups, and then to the glass cups, as what we see today. Therapy cups can also be made from **earthenware** and silicone materials that can withstand being exposed to elevated temperatures during the heating process.

> ### New Words and Expressions
>
> **alternative** /ɔːlˈtɜːnətɪv/ *adj.* offering or expressing a choice 替代的；备选的
> **e.g.** We had no alternative plan but to fire Gibson.
>
> **earthenware** /ˈɜːθənweə/ *n.* something made of clay that is baked so that it becomes hard 陶器
> **e.g.** Many sculptures were produced in earthenware.

New Words and Expressions

vacuum /ˈvækjʊəm/ *n.* a space that contains no air or other gas 真空

e.g. The dust is drawn into the vacuum cleaner.

myriad /ˈmɪrɪəd/ *n.* an extremely large number of things 无数，大量

e.g. Designs are available in a myriad of colors.

❸ Several other cultures used cupping therapy as a method to treat different ailments. The Chinese have been reported to use cupping during surgical procedures as a way to help divert the blood flow from the surgical site. American and European doctors have used cupping to treat more common ailments such as colds, chest infections, and congestion.

❹ Cupping therapy, also known as hijama therapy in some Arabic cultures, is a fascinating alternative form of medicine that has received mention in historical accounts dating from possibly 5,000 years ago. Chinese cupping therapy is often used in conjunction with more commonly known forms of traditional Chinese medicine treatments and methods such as acupuncture and acupressure.

❺ The basic idea behind cupping therapy is to place glass cups or silicone cups on the patient's skin to create a **vacuum**, so the blood is drawn to the surface of the skin in specific parts of the body that need healing. Traditional Chinese practitioners discuss different areas, or meridians, of the body that are used to transfer energy. They believe each body has 12 different meridians and treatment can be applied to each meridian for a **myriad** of reasons.

❻ Many athletes are known to use the cupping method as an alternative medicine. Some of these athletes include Michael Phelps and the USA Men's Olympic gymnastics team, as well as some members of the USA Track and Field team.

7 It is a very common practice among athletes and is considered an effective treatment to increase motion and soothe sore and tired muscles. The increased blood flow to the treated areas helps to promote muscle healing. It is especially helpful when the patient is competing in a sport such as swimming, gymnastics, or track and field because they are constantly using these muscles. Increasing the blood flow will help loosen these muscles and improve the range of motion these athletes have.

8 Many athletes use other methods in combination with the cupping method such as manual therapy, **sauna** and steaming, and cold therapy compression. It is a way for these athletes to release the muscles and tendons that they are constantly using in their sport. It is also beneficial when combined with massage therapy and has been reported to help athletes considerably with their pain management during training and events.

9 Three different traditional cupping methods have been used, including dry cupping, wet cupping, and massage cupping. For example, dry cupping produces a low amount of pressure. The cups are better suited for use on the softer tissue so that a secure and tight seal is allowed against the skin. The skin may also be lubricated so that the cups can be moved around from one area to a larger area. Wet cupping is a form of bloodletting and is used to remove stagnant blood, expel heat, and provide pain relief. It is imperative that the environment in which the wet

New Words and Expressions

sauna /ˈsɔːnə/ *n.* (a period of time spent in) a room or small building, often with wood attached to the walls, which is heated to a high temperature, usually with steam 桑拿浴；桑拿浴室

e.g. It was really hot in the sauna.

New Words and Expressions

sterilize /ˈsterɪlaɪz/ v. to kill the bacteria in or on something 灭菌；消毒
e.g. Sulphur (硫黄) is used to sterilize equipment.

cupping therapy is performed is clean and **sterilized** to prevent infection to the treatment sites.

(647 words)

(Source: Alin. 2019. The Secrets Behind Cupping Therapy. 01–10. From Cupping Resource website.)

Task One

Decide whether the following statements are true (T) or false (F) according to the text.

1. _____ Cupping therapy is incompatible with other kinds of Chinese medicine.

2. _____ Therapy cups made of silicone may melt in high temperatures during heating.

3. _____ Cupping therapy is not as widely recognized as acupuncture.

4. _____ A small amount of air should be injected into cups to stimulate blood to the surface.

5. _____ Ointment (软膏) can be applied on the skin to ensure the smooth movement of cupping in different areas.

Task Two

Fill in the blanks with the words given below. Change their forms if necessary.

alternative	evolve	withstand	divert	fascinating
lubricate	loosen	soothe	conjunction	imperative

1. Textbooks are designed to be used in _____ with classroom teaching.

2. Madagascar is the most _____ place I have ever been to; it's amazing!

3. Mineral oils are used to _____ machinery.

4. She failed to _____ the stresses and strains of public life.

5. New ways to treat arthritis may provide a(n) _____ to painkillers.

6. It uses therapy animals to _____ nervous passengers.

7. Birds are widely believed to have _____ from dinosaurs.

8. It is _____ to continue the treatment for at least two months.

9. He told her not to _____ the seat belt when he drove.

10. We _____ a plane to rescue 100 passengers.

Task Three

Paraphrase the following sentences from Text A.

1. The Chinese have been reported to use cupping during surgical procedures as a way to help divert the blood flow from the surgical site. (Para. 3)

_____

_____

_____

_____

2. Increasing the blood flow will help loosen these muscles and improve the range of motion these athletes have. (Para. 7)

_____

_____

_____

_____

3. The cups are better suited for use on the softer tissue so that a secure and tight seal is allowed against the skin. (Para. 9)

_____

_____

_____

_____

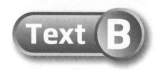

Benefits of Chinese Cupping

New Words and Expressions

infirmity /ɪnˈfɜːmɪtɪ/ *n.* weakness or illness over a long period（长期的）体弱；生病

e.g. We all fear disability or infirmity.

auxiliary /ɔːɡˈzɪljərɪ/ *adj.* supplementary; constituting a reserve 辅助的

e.g. The government's first concern was to expand the auxiliary forces.

❶ "Acupuncture and cupping, more than half of the ills cured" is a famous Chinese saying, supporting traditional Chinese medicine. Traditional Chinese medicine brings to mind acupuncture and the use of natural herbs as healing remedies. Cupping is a lesser-known treatment that is also part of Oriental medicine, one that can provide an especially pleasant experience. One of the earliest documentations of cupping can be found in the work titled *A Handbook of Prescriptions for Emergencies*, which was written by a Taoist herbalist by the name of Ge Hong and which dates all the way back to AD 300. An even earlier Chinese documentation, 3,000 years old, recommended cupping for the treatment of pulmonary tuberculosis. In both Eastern and Western cultures, cupping evolved from shamanistic (萨满教式的) practices that held the belief that illnesses and **infirmities** can be sucked out of the body.

❷ Cupping was established as an official therapeutic practice in the 1950s across hospitals in China after research conducted by Chinese and Soviet Union acupuncturists confirmed cupping's effectiveness. Prior to the 1950s, cupping had also been practiced as an **auxiliary** method in traditional Chinese surgery. In recent years, cupping has been growing in popularity, with celebrities like Gwyneth Paltrow, Jennifer Aniston, David Arquette, and the athlete Michael Phelps drawing public attention to the traditional benefits of Chinese cupping therapy techniques.

3 Though news outlets were quick to criticize celebrities chasing the newest medical therapies and techniques, recent studies have shown cupping's effectiveness in reducing pain intensity and providing positive short-term benefits.

4 The cupping therapist may **swab** alcohol onto the bottom of the cup, then light it, and put the cup immediately against the skin. Suction can also be created by placing an inverted cup over a small flame, or by using an alcohol-soaked cotton pad over an **insulating** material (like leather) to protect the skin, then lighting the pad, and placing an empty cup over the flame to extinguish it. Flames are never used near the skin and are not lit throughout the process of cupping, but rather are a means to create the heat that causes the suction within the small cups.

5 Once the suction has occurred, the cups can be gently moved across the skin (often referred to as "gliding cupping"). Medical massage oils are sometimes applied to improve movement of the glass cups along the skin. The suction in the cups causes the skin and superficial muscle layer to be lightly drawn into the cup. Cupping is much like the inverse of massage—rather than applying pressure to muscles, it uses gentle pressure to pull them upward. For most patients,

New Words and Expressions

swab /swɒb/ *v.* to apply (usually a liquid) to a surface 涂抹
e.g. The nurse swabbed the wound with something.

insulating /'ɪnsjʊleɪtɪŋ/ *adj.* preventing heat, sound, electricity from passing through 起隔热（或隔音、绝缘）作用的
e.g. We mentioned the insulating effect of snow.

New Words and Expressions

stagnation /stæɡˈneɪʃn/ *n.* no more development or progress 停滞
e.g. Stagnation in home sales is holding back economic recovery.

lymph /lɪmf/ *n.* a clear liquid that transports useful substances around the body, and carries waste matter such as unwanted bacteria away from body tissue in order to prevent infection 淋巴
e.g. Then, he was given the news that the cancer had spread to his lymph nodes.

phlegm /flem/ *n.* the thick substance that forms in the nose and throat 痰
e.g. His throat congested with phlegm.

this is a particularly relaxing and relieving sensation. Once sucked, the cups are generally left in place for about ten minutes while the patient relaxes. This is similar to the practice of *Tuina*, a traditional Chinese medicine massage technique that targets acupuncture points as well as painful body parts, and is well-known to provide relief through pressure.

❻ The old Chinese medical maxim "Where there's **stagnation**, there will be pain. Remove the stagnation, and you remove the pain" holds that pain results from the congestion, stagnation, and blockage of *qi* or vital energy, vital fluids, **lymph**, **phlegm**, and blood. If pain is the essence of disease, suffering is a result of obstructed or irregular flow in the body. Chinese cupping is therefore a method of breaking up the blockage to restore the body's natural flow of energy.

(567 words)

(Source: Rushall, K. 2019. Benefits of Chinese Cupping. 12–02. From Pacific College website.)

Task

Text B has six paragraphs. Choose the correct summary for each of them from the list below.

List of Paragraph Summaries

1.	Like *Tuina*, sucked cups with medical oils slowly move back and forth on the skin and gently pull muscles upward, giving patients a sense of relief.
2.	Cupping received mixed praise and criticism.

3.	Cupping has gained great popularity among famous figures for its therapeutic effect.
4.	The correlation between pain and cupping is deeply based on Chinese philosophy.
5.	Even not well-known around the world, cupping still boasts a profound history since ancient times in China and the West.
6.	There are several ways of creating the suction in the cups.

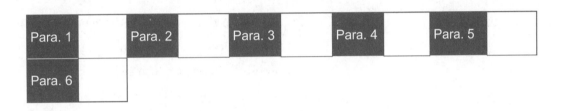

Para. 1		Para. 2		Para. 3		Para. 4		Para. 5	

Para. 6	

Post-reading

A Cupping Therapy Overview

❶ Cupping therapy originated in China. It is a practice that involves briefly applying rounded inverted cups to certain parts of the body using a vacuum effect. Some **proponents** suggest that the drawing of the skin inside the cups increases blood flow to the area.

❷ Long used in traditional Chinese medicine and other ancient healing systems, cupping has gained considerable popularity in recent years

> **New Words and Expressions**
>
> **proponent** /prə'pəʊnənt/ *n.* a person who speaks publicly in support of a particular idea or plan of action 支持者；建议者
> **e.g.** He is one of the leading proponents of capital punishment.

flammable /ˈflæməbl/ *adj.* burning easily 易燃的；可燃的

e.g. Caution! This solvent is highly flammable.

puncture /ˈpʌŋktʃə/ *v.* to make a small hole by a sharp point 在……上扎孔

e.g. She was taken to the hospital with a punctured lung.

among athletes. For instance, the swimmer Michael Phelps had the therapy in preparation for the 2016 Summer Olympics.

❸   In traditional Chinese medicine, cupping is said to stimulate the flow of vital energy and blood, and to help correct any imbalances arising from illness or injury. It's sometimes combined with acupuncture and *Tuina*, other therapies said to promote the flow of energy.

How Does Cupping Therapy Work?

❹   To create the suction inside the cups, the practitioner creates a vacuum by placing a **flammable** substance (such as herbs, alcohol, and/or paper) inside each cup and then ignites that substance. Next, the practitioner places the cup on the body. During a typical cupping treatment, between three and seven cups are placed on the body.

❺   Today, many practitioners use a manual or electric pump to create the vacuum, or use self-suctioning cupping sets. After the cups are in place, they are usually removed after five to ten minutes. Some practitioners may practice "flash" cupping.

❻   Some practitioners apply massage oil or cream and then attach silicone cups, sliding them around the body rhythmically for a massage-like effect.

❼   In a procedure known as "wet cupping", the skin is **punctured** prior to treatment. This causes blood to flow out of the punctures during the cupping procedure, which is thought to clear toxins from the body.

Benefits

8   To date, there is a lack of high-quality scientific research to support the use of cupping to treat any health condition. For instance, a research review in 2011 sized up seven trials testing cupping in people with pain (such as low back pain); results showed that most of the studies were of poor quality.

9   In another research review published in 2017, scientists analyzed 11 studies that tested the use of cupping by athletes. The review's authors concluded that no explicit recommendation could be made for or against the use of cupping in athletes and that further studies were needed.

10   Some studies did show that cupping improved **perceptions** of pain and disability and had favorable effects on the range of motion compared to no cupping.

11   Although cupping is sometimes recommended to increase flexibility in athletes, a small study published in *The Journal of Sports Rehabilitation* in 2018 found no change in hamstring (绳肌腱) flexibility after a seven-minute cupping session using four cups. Study participants were NCAA Division III college soccer players without symptoms.

Possible Side Effects

12   Cupping may cause pain, swelling, burns, dizziness, lightheadedness, fainting, sweating, skin **pigmentation**, and/or nausea. Cupping also leaves round purple marks or circular bruises on the skin; these marks may begin to fade after several days but can remain for two to three

New Words and Expressions

perception /pə'sepʃn/ *n.* the way one notices things, especially with the senses 知觉；感知
e.g. The visual perception comes from observation of physical movement.

pigmentation /ˌpɪgmən'teɪʃn/ *n.* the presence of pigments in skin, hair, leaves, etc. that causes them to be a particular color; natural coloring 色素沉着；天然颜色
e.g. I have a skin disorder which destroys the pigmentation in my skin.

New Words and Expressions

hemophilia /ˌhiːməˈfɪlɪə/ *n.* a medical condition in which a person's blood does not thicken or clot properly when he or she is injured, so he or she continues bleeding 血友病
e.g. The family apparently suffered from a very rare form of hemophilia.

high-profile /ˌhaɪˈprəʊfaɪl/ *adj.* receiving a lot of attention and discussion on television or in newspapers 经常出镜的；高姿态的
e.g. He is a high-profile lawyer.

weeks. Scars and burns have been known to occur after cupping.

⓭　Cupping shouldn't be done on areas where the skin is broken, irritated, or inflamed, or over arteries, veins, or any fractures.

⓮　People who are pregnant, children, older adults, and people with certain health conditions (such as cancer, organ failure, **hemophilia**, edema, blood disorders, and some types of heart disease) are among those who shouldn't have cupping. People taking blood-thinning medication also shouldn't try cupping.

⓯　The practitioner should follow standard infection control practices and safety precautions to protect against the transmission of diseases (such as hepatitis).

Conclusion

⓰　After seeing **high-profile** athletes and celebrities sport the characteristic round purple marks, someone may find it tempting to try cupping, but there's currently a lack of research on cupping. If you're still thinking of trying it, be sure to consult your doctor before beginning treatment.

(640 words)

(Source: Wong, C. 2020. Holistic Health: Cupping Therapy Overview, Benefits, and Side Effects. 04–06. From Verywell Health website.)

Your reading time: _____ mins

Your reading rate: _____ words/min

Task

Read the text as quickly as you can and then choose the best answer to each question.

1. Which of the following statements is true about cupping methods according to the text?

   A. Materials that catch fire easily should be avoided so as to protect skin from injury.

   B. Cups can be gently moved across the skin at regular intervals.

   C. It's advisable to refrain from placing cups too hurriedly.

   D. Wet cups need clear water to rinse skin wounds before punctures.

2. What do we know about the benefits of cupping?

   A. Cupping is more often used in comparison with other traditional Chinese medicine techniques.

   B. Trials involving athletes who have used cupping present solid evidence about its therapeutic effect.

   C. Researchers strongly recommend cupping because it makes athletes' muscles more flexible.

   D. The potential medical benefits of cupping need further exploration.

3. Which person mentioned below is suitable for cupping?

   A. A teenager who is sensitive about her beautiful appearance.

   B. A senior citizen whose left leg was broken days ago.

   C. An office lady who often stays up late for work.

   D. An athlete whose skin is red and swollen after sunburn.

4. What does "sport" in Para. 16 mean?

   A. To play happily.

   B. To exercise.

   C. To detect.

   D. To display.

5. Which of the following statements is true according to the text?

   A. Cupping is still a dangerous therapy that needs more study.

   B. Cupping can be applied to a variety of patients except for those with incurable diseases.

   C. You'd better seek advice from medical professionals before trying cupping.

D. The negative effect of cupping can be eliminated when it is used with other medicine.

Your comprehension rate: _____ %

Additional Reading

A Review of Clinical Studies on Cupping Therapy

New Words and Expressions

complementary /ˌkɒmplɪˈmentrɪ/ *adj.* (of two or more different things) combing in such a way as to form a complete whole or to enhance or emphasize each other's qualities 互补的

e.g. The school's approach must be complementary to that of the parents.

❶   Cupping therapy is a traditional therapeutic technique that is used as a **complementary** and alternative treatment worldwide. The categories of cupping therapy are becoming more diverse; however, it can generally be classified into retained cupping, moving cupping, flashing cupping, blood-letting puncture cupping, and needle-retaining cupping. According to the results of our previous studies, cupping therapy may have a significant benefit in the treatment of pain-related conditions, herpes zoster (带状疱疹), facial paralysis, and cervical spondylosis (颈椎病).

❷   It is widely believed that it is the temperature and the continuous vacuum generated during cupping therapy that make an impact on local skin. This continuous vacuum may stretch the skin and underlying tissue, induce vascular recruitment, and cause the capillaries to dilate and break. Regional stimulation causes a micro-environmental change in vivo and leads to secretion of chemical signals. Furthermore, these regional chemical signals interact with each other, eventually resulting in a systemic effect. Dr Lowe indicated in his review that cupping therapy may have **antioxidant**, antiinflammatory, metabolic regulative, and immunomodulatory (免疫调节的) effects in animal and human systems.

❸　Investigating the mechanism and impact of cupping therapy may help **elucidate** its local and systemic effects. However, high-quality clinical evidence that can explain the key elements and mechanism of cupping therapy is still lacking. Professor Lee assessed five systematic reviews and came to a conclusion that reduction of pain may be the only therapeutic effect of cupping. However, this indication is not well proven as well. Given the variation in the findings of previous studies, it is necessary to critically evaluate and summarize the existing clinical evidence for obtaining a clearer picture of the mechanism and therapeutic effect of cupping therapy. In this review, the key elements that determine the efficacy of cupping therapy were summarized and evaluated based on evidence in the currently available literature. The results of this review would provide practitioners with a clearer direction regarding the use of cupping

New Words and Expressions

antioxidant /ˌæntɪˈɒksɪdənt/ n. a substance like vitamin C that removes dangerous molecules such as free radicals from the body 抗氧化物
e.g. The natural antioxidant found in red wine may protect cells from damage.

elucidate /ɪˈluːsɪdeɪt/ v. to make something clearer by explaining it more fully 阐明；解释
e.g. He elucidated a point of grammar.

therapy in clinical practice. The aim of this review was to identify the possible mechanisms behind cupping therapy by utilizing an evidence-based approach, and to explore its possible regional and systemic effects in the human body.

Methods

④ We searched six electronic databases and four online trial registries for articles published up to January 1, 2020. The methodological qualities of controlled studies were assessed using the National Institute for Clinical Excellence methodology checklist, the Newcastle-Ottawa Scale, and the Cochrane risk of bias tool. Characteristic statistical description and qualitative summary of results were used for data analysis.

Results

⑤ 38 studies (37 full texts and 1 abstract) were included in this study. Due to the clinical **heterogeneity** among the studies, we could not conduct a meta-analysis. The results showed that the key factors that contribute to the efficacy of cupping therapy are negative pressure and temperature. Cupping therapy mainly causes local and systemic changes in hemodynamics, immune regulation, metabolism, and pain relief.

Discussion

⑥ We divided the included studies into two categories; some trials explored the elements that may contribute to the efficacy of cupping, whereas others showed what physical changes would occur after treatment. According to the results of the studies in the first category, negative pressure during cupping treatment may play a more critical role than temperature in the curative effect of cupping therapy. However, it must be noted for negative pressure because the concept of "the higher, the better" is not always true.

Conclusion

⑦ We identified negative pressure as the key element behind cupping therapy. Cupping therapy may cause redistribution of oxygen at the cupping site and in neighboring tissues, thereby inducing a therapeutic effect by increasing regional blood flow. It may also induce metabolic change, immunomodulation (免疫调节), and neuromodulation (神经调节). However, additional rigorous clinical research needs to be conducted to further clarify the mechanism behind cupping therapy.

(619 words)

[Source: Anon. 2020. Key Elements that Determine the Efficacy of Cupping Therapy: A Bibliometric Analysis and Review of Clinical Studies. *Journal of Traditional Chinese Medical Sciences*, *7*(4): 345-354.]

Task

Read the text carefully and then complete the statements with appropriate words.

1. The traditionally therapeutic effect of cupping means it is _____ to other treatments.

2. The _____ culture of America, to some extent, comes from its immigrants of various backgrounds.

3. The _____ impact of cupping therapy lies in its relief of painful diseases.

4. An investigation into the working theory of cupping therapy may _____ its local and systemic effects.

5. To _____ the existing clinical evidence is vital to obtain a clear understanding of the therapeutic effect of cupping.

6. Employers must consider all candidates impartially and without _____.

7. Some experiments were conducted to look into the elements that may affect the _____ of cupping.

8. The results revealed that negative pressure and temperature were the key factors that contributed to the _____ effect of cupping therapy.

9. Nothing—except the prospect for promotion—would _____ me to take the job.

10. Red wine helps to _____ and widen blood vessels with larger space.

Unit 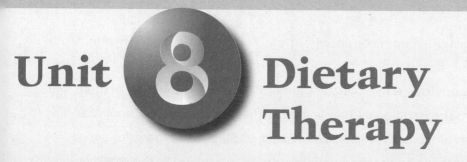 Dietary Therapy

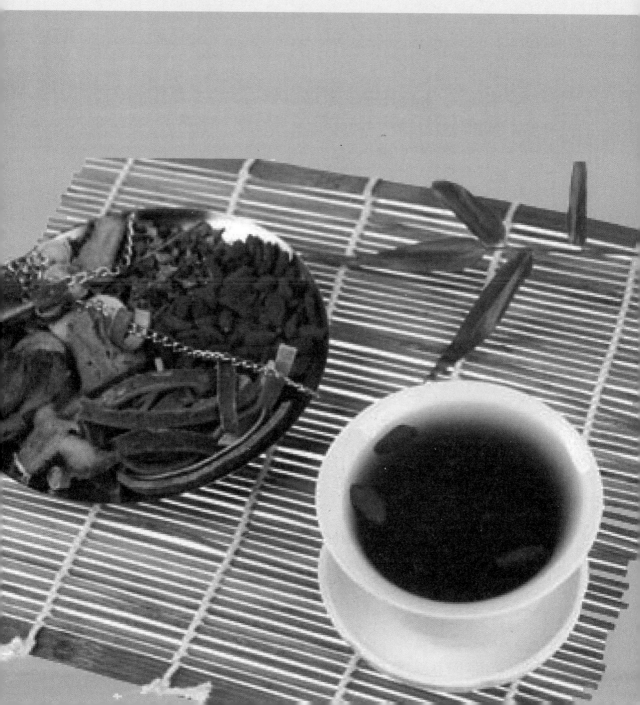

Pre-reading

Food is consumed daily for energy, strength, disease prevention, and health maintenance. An incorrect diet can cause exhaustion and fatigue as well as weight gain and skin conditions. A diet therapy promotes a balanced selection of foods vital for good health. The traditional Chinese dietary therapy involves the understanding of the properties of foods, their effects on health, and the use of foods for preventing and treating illnesses. It is also recommended to eat, according to the characteristics of each season, to keep healthy. In traditional Chinese medicine, there are no distinct differences between food and medicine. In other words, food itself can sometimes be all the medicine you need.

Do you know what a traditional Chinese dietary therapy is? What's the magical effect of eating seasonal foods? How do the foods we eat help keep us healthy? How does a Chinese dietary therapy work for children? To find out the answers, let's explore the journey with food.

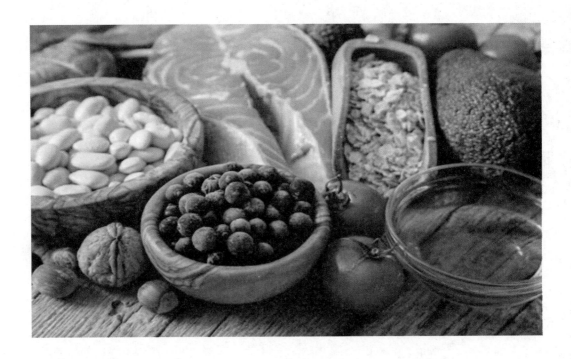

In-reading

Text A

Chinese Dietary Therapy

❶ Traditional Chinese medicine is a holistic and comprehensive health care system that views the body in accordance with nature. It puts the utmost importance on lifestyle choices and nutrition, and if these fail to bring the body into balance, it is time to look into herbs and acupuncture. In TCM, there are no distinct differences between food and medicine, meaning that food itself can sometimes be all the medicine you need. Food is viewed as a powerful tool to help create and maintain wellness.

❷ The basis of healthy eating in regards to TCM is filling most of the diet with fresh foods that are free from chemicals, preservatives, and over-processing. These foods are seen as the most vital, full of *qi*.

❸ Vegetables should be cooked only lightly to preserve beneficial enzymes and vitamins. People should eat according to their particular **constitution**, with the largest meal of the day in the morning. Beans and grains should be soaked

> **New Words and Expressions**
>
> **constitution** /ˌkɒnstɪˈtjuːʃn/ *n.* the general state of someone's health 体质，体格
> e.g. He has a very strong constitution.

New Words and Expressions

optimal /ˈɒptɪml/ *adj.* the best or most suitable 最佳的，最优的

e.g. We have found that our workers reach their optimal level of performance around 11 am.

and properly cooked to allow for easy digestion. Not only is a healthy diet integral to **optimal** health, but it is crucial to get physical and mental exercise as well as rest.

❹　According to Chinese medicine, every food and herb has a nature, flavor, and organ system/meridian associated with it. The nature describes the effect of the foods (or herbs) on the temperature of the body, while the flavor describes the taste.

❺　Instead of viewing meals as a breakdown of proteins, carbohydrates (sugars), and fats, Chinese dietary therapy utilizes the flavors and natures of foods as a guide to a well-balanced meal. Learning how to utilize the natures and flavors of foods and herbs is really where the true healing capacity of this diet lays.

❻　There is also the belief that the seasons have a profound impact upon our well-being, and eating according to the seasons can have great impacts on our health. We are immensely influenced by changes in the climate and we should learn to live and eat in balance with those changes.

❼　Chinese diet therapy also focuses on a mentality that "like treats like". For example, if a woman had a particularly heavy menstrual cycle and was feeling fatigued, eating some extra red meat or foods high in iron can help. If someone was struggling with pain in his or her joints, some bone broth can do the trick. Also foods that resemble parts of the body are often used according to a traditional practice to help support that specific part: walnuts for the brain, pomegranates (石榴) for women's health.

8 There is a lot to learn when it comes to Chinese medicine and the Five Elements, but even learning and **incorporating** the basics into your everyday life can have profound impacts. The main lesson here is to observe your body and its patterns to learn what it needs to find balance. Some simple ideas are that if you are feeling overheated, eat some cooling cucumbers; feeling **bloated** or having edema, cut down on your salt intake. A great way to incorporate healing foods and herbs into your diet is to make congee!

9 If you want to go deeper into Chinese dietary therapy, it is advised that you see a Chinese medicine practitioner or acupuncturist. They will be able to figure out the pattern differentiation of your current constitution. This will usually be an explanation of where the body is out of balance in regards to the Five Elements or organ systems (heart / small intestine, spleen/stomach, lung / large intestine, kidney/bladder, liver/ gallbladder).

10 Once you have this information, you will be able to make more informed decisions of what flavors and natures of foods can nurture your body best.

> **New Words and Expressions**
>
> **incorporate** /ɪnˈkɔːpəreɪt/ *v.* to make into a whole or make part of a whole; to include 吸收；包含
> e.g. Many of your suggestions have been incorporated in the plan.
>
> **bloated** /ˈbləʊtɪd/ *adj.* overfilled and extended with liquid, gas, food, etc.（身体部位）肿起的；饮食过度的
> e.g. Diners do not want to leave the table feeling bloated.

(607 words)

(Source: Cangeloso, L. 2018. Chinese Dietary Therapy. 09–06. From Wild Earth Acupuncture website.)

Task One

Decide whether the following statements are true (T) or false (F) according to the text.

1. _____   If you find certain parts of your body out of balance, probably it is time to turn to herbs or acupuncture.

2. _____   According to traditional Chinese medicine, there are no real differences between food and medicine, and many herbs are considered a kind of food which could be eaten in daily life.

3. _____   If a woman feels tired, eating more vegetables and fruits can help.

4. _____   It is a good way to put all kinds of herbs into your porridge if you feel sick.

5. _____   To determine the appropriate foods to consume, it is essential that you first consult a traditional Chinese medicine practitioner, who will make recommendations based on how your organs are functioning.

Task Two

Fill in the blanks with the words and phrase given below. Change their forms if necessary.

in accordance with	integral	holistic	optimal	breakdown
congee	incorporate	bloated	resemble	fatigue

1. Think about areas that interest you and where you can add value. Then, go ahead and pitch yourself as a(n) _____ part of the team.

2. China is trying to make _____ use of educational resources so that rural and underdeveloped areas will get more support.

3. He was always neatly and quietly dressed _____ his age and station.

4. I felt _____ from eating too much yesterday.

5. A regular breakfast can consist of soybeans, an egg, a bowl of _____, corn, a sweet potato, meat, and two kinds of fruit.

6. No computer is as smart as a human being with a(n) _____ point of view.

7. For example, universities could _____ Individual Development Plan into their graduate curricula to help students discuss, plan, prepare for, and achieve their long-term career goals.

8. The boys _____ in that they both have ginger hair and round faces.

9. He thinks that breaking with tradition leads to all sorts of serious social problems, even the _____ of the fabric of society.

10. Driver _____ was to blame for the accident.

Task Three

Paraphrase the following sentences from Text A.

1. Traditional Chinese medicine is a holistic and comprehensive health care system that views the body in accordance with nature. (Para. 1)

_____

_____

_____

_____

2. There is also the belief that the seasons have a profound impact upon our well-being, and eating according to the seasons can have great impacts on our health. (Para. 6)

_____

_____

_____

_____

3. This will usually be an explanation of where the body is out of balance in regards to the Five Elements or organ systems (heart / small intestine, spleen/ stomach, lung / large intestine, kidney/bladder, liver/gallbladder). (Para. 9)

_____

_____

_____

_____

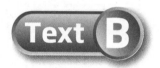

Seasonal Foods in Accordance with TCM

❶ The COVID-19 pandemic has more than changed the way we live our lives—it has also affected the way we eat. As most of us are spending more time at home, we've all been cooking more, craving comfort foods and even becoming more aware of the impact of healthy eating on the immune system.

❷ According to TCM philosophies, what we eat and drink is one of the keys to staying healthy. It's believed that if we consume foods that are similar in nature to the external environment, our bodies will be able to adapt to seasonal changes better, thus maintaining harmonious *qi* and improving our overall well-being. To master the technique of using seasonal foods as medicines to boost immunity, it's important to understand the 24 solar terms. It's an ancient Chinese lunar calendar that indicates seasonal changes, best agricultural practices as well as wellness tips based on the sun's position in the **ecliptic** throughout the year.

❸ Known as the first solar term of the Chinese lunar calendar, *Li Chun* represents the beginning of spring—a time of rebirth and **revival**. Springtime is associated with "wood" in the Chinese Five Elements Theory, which suggests that human bodies, just like crops, will experience a new phase of "growth" that we should nourish our yang energy more for better health.

❹ The wood element also corresponds to our liver—an organ which governs the overall *qi* and our emotions. During spring, we should increase our intake of dates, spinach, onion, soybean products, radishes, sour citrus fruits, and avoid eating fats and highly-seasoned foods to **detoxify** the liver for a smooth flow of *qi* and better emotional health.

❺ Signifying the end of spring and the arrival of summer, *Li Xia* is the peak time to harvest crops. The weather is becoming warmer, and thunderstorms will occur more frequently too. Summer belongs to "fire" in the Chinese Five Elements Theory, which symbolizes humans' abundant energy in hot summer days. It tells the importance of nourishing our body (especially our heart) with foods that carry yin (cold) energy to keep ourselves cool and ease heat

New Words and Expressions

glutinous /'gluːtɪnəs/ *adj.* having the sticky properties 黏的；胶质的

e.g. Eating *yuanxiao* (sweet dumplings made of glutinous rice flour) is one of the special traditions of the Lantern Festival.

exhaustion symptoms such as heavy sweating, heart palpitations, insomnia, and anxiety.

6　Fresh vegetables, including lotus root, cucumber, celery, and fruits such as strawberries, watermelons, and bananas are top food recommendations for summer. It's also good to have more bitter greens such as bitter melon and kale.

7　Though the heat from summer still stays in the air right now, autumn has officially begun. *Li Qiu* is the first solar term of the new season, which reflects the beginning of cooler months and a transitional period into a drier climate.

8　Autumn is associated with "metal" in the Chinese Five Elements Theory. It correlates with our lung system and the color white, when Chinese people often consume foods in white color such as snow fungus, lotus seed, and lily bulb to nourish the lungs. Keeping our lungs healthy to fend off respiratory viruses has become particularly important at times like this, so it's advisable to consume not only more white foods, but also foods that can help hydrate the body and boost our metabolism such as honey, **glutinous** rice, pineapple, and pear.

9　*Li Dong* signals the beginning of winter, in which the season is all about rest and restoring our energy. Winter belongs to "water" in the Chinese Five Elements Theory, meaning we should not disturb our yang energy and nourish our yin energy more, to build strength before stepping into the warmer season, spring.

10　In TCM, winter corresponds to our kidneys,

and it's believed that good *qi* in the organ will keep the bones, brain, as well as reproductive and urinary systems healthy. During the cold season, we should consume an appropriate amount of fat and high-protein foods such as beef, eggs, dates, mushrooms, and glutinous rice to keep the body warm. It's also necessary to eat less salt to maintain the kidney's health and keep a certain amount of yin food intake for a balanced diet.

(664 words)

(Source: Yu, H. 2020. Seasonal Foods in Accordance with TCM. 08–11. From Tatlerasia website.)

Task

Text B has ten paragraphs. Choose the correct summary for each of them from the list below.

List of Paragraph Summaries

1.	We should eat foods that carry yin energy to nourish heart in summer.
2.	It is suggested to consume white food and nourish our lungs during this season.
3.	It begins a season of nourishing yin energy and builds strength before a warmer season.
4.	Some fresh vegetables, fruits, and bitter greens are recommended for this season.
5.	We should master the technique of using seasonal foods as medicines to boost our immunity.

6.	It signifies the beginning of cooler months.
7.	It is suggested to nourish our yang energy in springtime.
8.	It is important to keep the body warm and maintain the kidney's health.
9.	The COVID-19 pandemic has changed our way of eating.
10.	We should take food to detoxify the liver for a smooth flow of *qi*.

Para. 1		Para. 2		Para. 3		Para. 4		Para. 5	
Para. 6		Para. 7		Para. 8		Para. 9		Para. 10	

Post-reading

Healthy Eating in Traditional Chinese Medicine

New Words and Expressions

clan /klæn/ *n.* a group of families who are related to each other 宗族；部族
e.g. This clan was once very powerful, and easily dominated Ork society for a long time.

❶ The Chinese have their own answer to healthy eating, with concepts strongly related to traditional Chinese medicine. They are probably the most hard-core supporters of the saying "You are what you eat", regardless of whether they really follow that advice.

❷ The ancient **clans** of China, dating back to 2,200 BC, started to discover the different medical values of herbs while they were still hunting and gathering. Some foods relieved their illness, and some caused death. Over time, and in **concourse** with the growth of Chinese philosophy, medical theories were developed.

New Words and Expressions

concourse /ˈkɒŋkɔːs/ *n.* an act or process of coming together and merging 集合；合流
e.g. The great concourse of people seemed to have been similarly impressed.

❸ In traditional Chinese medicine, food is divided into five natures, respectively, cold, cool, neutral, warm, and hot. The nature of food is not determined by their actual temperature, but rather by what effects they have on a person's body after consumption. When a person continually eats one type of food, it creates an imbalance in his or her body, and affects his or her immune system. Thus, one of the keys in Chinese medicine is to keep our body "neutral".

❹ Foods that are warm and hot bring heat to our bodies—e.g. beef, coffee, ginger, hot chilies, and fried foods—while cold and cool foods cool down our bodies—think of salad, cheese, green tea, and beer. Neutral foods are foods like oil, rice, pork, and most kinds of fishes.

❺ A person who has too much heat in his or her body usually feels hot, sweats all the time, is grumpy, has a swollen tongue, or could be constipated. People who have too much cold in their bodies appear pale, have cold hands and feet, might feel weak, or have bad blood circulation. When this happens, we are advised to stop eating that kind of food.

❻ Like the Westerners, the Chinese divide tastes into five different kinds (*wuwei*): sour, bitter, sweet, spicy, and salty. But for the Chinese, these are more than just senses. In traditional Chinese medicine, each bite of foods sends the nutrition to corresponding organs: Sour food enters the liver, and helps stop sweating and ease coughing; salt enters the kidneys, and can drain, **purge**, and soften masses; bitter food enters the heart and the small intestine, and helps cool heat and dry any dampness; spicy food enters the lungs and the large intestine, and helps stimulate appetite; sweet food enters the stomach and spleen, and helps "lubricate" the body. Thus, it is important to have each flavor in the diet.

7 Does that mean to be healthy we just eat neutral food in all flavors? Not necessarily. "Food choices are affected by your body's construction, the season, and the place where you live," said Chan. The condition of the body could also be affected by age and sex. In other words, Chinese medical practitioners adapt their recommendations to different conditions.

8 One size does not fit all. Just like we all have different personalities, we also have different body constitutions. And just like you cannot communicate with all people in the same way, we cannot feed our bodies with the same food in the same way either.

9 A person with a lot of "dampness and phlegm" in his or her body tends to be overweight, might sweat a lot, and might have an oily face. This kind of people is usually more mild-tempered.

10 However, a person with a lot of "dampness and heat" is usually short-tempered and often presents with an oily face and acne breakouts.

This kind of people needs different foods to take away their dampness, which means sweets, while "lubricating" the body, might worsen the situation. Each type of food, depending on its nature, might better or worsen the situation.

⓫ The season and time of a year is another factor when it comes to food choices. For instance, spring is often wet and sticky in China, which means we need food that can take away the dampness in our body such as corn, white beans, and onion.

(652 words)

(Source: Lee, H.-S. 2019. Healthy Eating in Traditional Chinese Medicine. 01–18. From DW website.)

Your reading time: _____ mins

Your reading rate: _____ words/min

Task

Read the text as quickly as you can and then choose the best answer to each question.

1. If one feels very cold, which food is not suggested to eat?

    A. Coffee.

    B. Fried food.

    C. Beer.

D. Ginger.

2. Which food is suggested for wet and sticky spring in south China according to the text?

A. White beans.

B. Shrimp.

C. Tomatoes.

D. Pepper.

3. What is the suggested food therapy if one wants to stop sweating and ease coughing?

A. He or she could eat sweet foods.

B. He or she could eat sour foods.

C. He or she could eat salty foods.

D. He or she could eat spicy foods.

4. A person tends to be fatty, might sweat a lot, and might have an oily face. From the Chinese medical perspective, we could judge that _____.

A. this person is usually short-tempered

B. this person is usually mean-tempered

C. this person is usually mild-tempered

D. this person is usually bad-tempered

5. Chinese medical practitioners considered that food choices are not affected by _____.

A. the place where a person lives

B. a person's job

C. a person's body constitution

D. a person's age and sex

Your comprehension rate: _____ %

Additional Reading

Chinese Dietary Therapy for Children

❶ It is the Chinese medical understanding that the spleen and stomach are the organs of digestion and **assimilation**.

❷ The stomach is the vessel that holds the food and the spleen is the fire beneath that cooks the food and distributes it. Therefore, anything that disrupts the function of the spleen/stomach or the digestion is harmful to the body's energy.

❸ A child's digestive system is insufficient especially when they are under six years old because this is the average age when a person's digestion matures.

❹ An immature digestion combined with an inappropriate diet accounts for the most encountered **pediatric** complaints including: **colic**, ear infections, diarrhea, constipation, eczema, cough, common cold, swollen glands, hyperactivity, allergies, and asthma.

❺ Just like we teach children about the world (science, math, art, writing, etc.), they need our guidance about what to eat. No children can eat whatever they want and still remain entirely healthy. My six-year-old daughter is a perfect example! Unless I'm with her to supervise that she's eaten her healthy food, she'll eat sugary, salty, greasy, processed foods by default.

New Words and Expressions

assimilation /əˌsɪmɪˈleɪʃn/ *n.* the process of absorbing food into the tissue of a living organism 吸收
e.g. Poor assimilation of vitamins and nutrients can cause health problems.

pediatric /ˌpiːdɪˈætrɪk/ *adj.* of or relating to the medical care of children 小儿科的
e.g. He completed his pediatric residency at Stanford University Hospital.

colic /ˈkɒlɪk/ *n.* severe pain in the stomach and bowels suffered especially by babies（尤指婴儿的）急性腹痛，腹绞痛
e.g. The doctor said it was colic and that she would grow out of it.

❻ Regardless of the condition, most children's diseases should surround regulating and strengthening the digestion. Focusing on a child's gut health is of the utmost importance for their health. There are, of course, other lifestyle factors that attribute to disease which include: stress, lack of exercise, and chronic exposure to toxins, but today I will concentrate on food choices.

❼ Children should be fed more plant-based wholesome foods with a high percentage of vegetables, fruits, grains, and smaller amounts of meats, eggs, and dairy products. Animal products are heavier to digest due to their dense nutritional value but are still considered a valuable resource for a child's growth.

❽ The majority of food a child eats should be cooked because cooked and warmed food is easier for them to digest due to their immature digestion. Kids under six years old should not eat just cold and raw foods because their digestive system is not mature yet. Older kids can eat more salads and fresh fruits which are in season and local because they have more nutrients. Meanwhile, you may need to identify and address food allergies. Gluten, soy, dairy, eggs, wheat, and yeast are the usual suspects when food allergies are concerned.

❾ Of course, TCM considers the seasons when offering nutritional guidelines. Winter is a time for **hearty** and warm foods like **stews** including root vegetables, meats, and spices like ginger, chili pepper, **cinnamon**, **nutmeg**, and **scallions**; summer is a time for cooling foods like citrus, tofu, milk, lettuce, celery, mint, cucumber, and tomato. Cook lighter meals using methods like steaming and stir-frying. Our bodies are as dynamic as the seasons so we must try to eat accordingly.

⑩ Balancing the flavors and colors of foods supports overall health of our bodies by nourishing the different systems with nutrients they need to function optimally. For example, white foods (mushrooms, garlic, daikon radishes) will strengthen the immune system. Orange foods (carrots, sweet potatoes, papayas) prevent inflammation. Red foods (red peppers, tomatoes, cherries) improve the cardiovascular system. Yellow foods (bananas, lemons, pineapples) fortify skin elasticity. Purple foods (eggplants, grapes, purple cabbages) protect the nervous system. Green foods (kale, celery, cucumbers) detoxify the body.

⑪ As children grow, limiting sweets and dairy foods is very important for a child's health. These inappropriate foods would include but are not limited to: flavored yogurt, juice, fruit snacks, and ice cream (to name a few), which are usually a child's first choice when asking for a snack. The sweet flavor and often cold temperature of these foods hamper digestion.

⑫ Instead, opt for warm applesauce **sprinkled** with cinnamon for a snack; and rather than a cold sandwich for lunch, offer soup. As most moms agree, making up a lunch box can be challenging, but storing soup in a thermos and

---

New Words and Expressions

sprinkle /ˈsprɪŋkl/ *v.* to scatter the liquid or powder over something 撒；用……点缀

e.g. She sprinkled sugar over the strawberries.

having fruits and vegetables available will make a difference.

(643 words)

(Source: Anon. 2019. Chinese Dietary Therapy for Children. 12–08. From Rose Wellness website.)

Task

Read the text carefully and then complete the statements with appropriate words.

1. The development of national culture goes side by side with the _____ of foreign culture.
2. As parents, we need to _____ children to eat the healthy food, far away from the junk food.
3. A child should eat cooked food because it is easy for them to digest due to their _____ digestion.
4. Do not undertake strenuous exercise for a few hours after a meal to allow food to _____.
5. Anyone who does not believe that smoking is an addiction has never been a _____ smoker.
6. _____ the meat with salt and place it in the pan.
7. Experts have linked this condition to a build-up of _____ in the body.
8. Flavored yogurt, juice, fruit snacks, and ice cream, a child's first choice when asking for a snack, are _____ to children's digestion.
9. The search was _____ by terrible weather conditions.
10. They _____ for more holiday instead of more pay.